Self Empower

USING

SELF-COACHING, NEUROADAPTABILITY,

AND AYURVEDA

Robert Keith Wallace, PhD, Samantha Wallace, Ted Wallace, MS

ISBN 978-1-7357401-1-9

Library of Congress Control Number: 2021906485

DharmaPublications.com

Dharma Publications, Fairfield, IA

To Our Very Dear Children and Grandchildren

OTHER BOOKS BY

Robert Keith Wallace, Samantha Wallace, and Ted Wallace

Trouble in Paradise
How to Deal with People Who Push Your Buttons
Using Total Brain Coaching
Robert Keith Wallace, PhD, Samantha Wallace,
Ted Wallace, MS

The Coherence Code
How to Maximize Your Performance and Success in Business
For Individuals, Teams, and Organizations
Robert Keith Wallace, PhD, Ted Wallace, MS,
Samantha Wallace

Total Brain Coaching
A Holistic System of Effective Habit Change
For the Individual, Team, and Organization
Ted Wallace, MS, Robert Keith Wallace, PhD,
Samantha Wallace

The Rest and Repair Diet
Heal Your Gut, Improve Your Physical and Mental Health,
and Lose Weight
Robert Keith Wallace, PhD, Samantha Wallace,
Andrew Stenberg, MA, Jim Davis, DO, with Alexis Farley

Gut Crisis
How Diet, Probiotics, and Friendly Bacteria
Help You Lose Weight and Heal Your Body and Mind
Robert Keith Wallace, PhD, Samantha Wallace

Dharma Parenting
Understand Your Child's Brilliant Brain for Greater
Happiness, Health, Success, and Fulfillment
Robert Keith Wallace, PhD, Frederick Travis, PhD

Quantum Golf
The Path to Golf Mastery
REVISED Second Edition
Kjell Enhager, Robert Keith Wallace, PhD, Samantha Wallace

The Maya of Beauty
A Friendly Introduction to Ayurveda,
Essential Oil Skincare, and Makeup for Real People
Samantha Wallace, Robert Keith Wallace, PhD

An Introduction to Transcendental Meditation
Improve Your Brain Functioning, Create Ideal Health,
and Gain Enlightenment Naturally, Easily, Effortlessly
Robert Keith Wallace, PhD, Lincoln Akin Norton

Transcendental Meditation
A Scientist's Journey to Happiness, Health, and Peace
Robert Keith Wallace, PhD

The Neurophysiology of Enlightenment
How the Transcendental Meditation and TM-Sidhi Program
Transform the Functioning of the Human Body
Robert Keith Wallace, PhD

Maharishi Ayurveda and Vedic Technology
Creating Ideal Health for the Individual and World
Robert Keith Wallace, PhD

The Coherence Effect
Tapping into the Laws of Nature that Govern Health,
Happiness, and Higher Brain Functioning
Robert Keith Wallace, PhD, Jay B. Marcus,
Christopher S. Clark, MD

CONTENTS

FOREWORD

Every winter a convergence of natural forces creates some of the largest and most dangerous waves in the world. Spawned from storms in the Gulf of Alaska, monstrous waves arise with furious strength, at Mavericks, a beach south of San Francisco. Up to 60-foot waves are a result of unusual undersea topography, water depth, temperature, tides, and wind—so strong that they register on seismic instruments 30 miles away at UC Berkeley.

Only highly skilled and experienced surfers in peak condition are able to take on such a challenge. The attempt to ride Mavericks' treacherous waves requires a delicate balance of brain neurochemicals to help attune them to the power of nature.

In business, too, even strong, intelligent leaders face powerful waves of change, especially when dealing with the complex convergence of Volatile, Uncertain, Complex, and Ambiguous forces—VUCA. Too often they attempt to control these waves rather than learning the subtleties of riding them.

My professional specialty is Adaptive Leadership and Business Agility and I work with executives at some of the top companies in the US, Australia, and all over the world. I have been an Adjunct Instructor and Professor for over 50 years and currently teach at the University of California at Berkeley. Today's adaptive leaders must be able to perceive and understand what others do not, and have the courage and clarity to lead companies through unpredictable and uncomfortable challenges. The hallmark of an adaptive leader is to respond creatively and effectively where others don't even notice possible threats. These leaders create a network of collaborative multidisciplinary teams who are accountable for each other's productivity and are united by a common purpose.

Improving your life starts with changing your mindset and your habits. Self Empower presents a set of remarkable neuroadaptability tools that can help anyone become more energetic, more flexible, more self-determined, and self-sufficient. These tools help you understand who you really are and how you can improve your ability to learn faster and increase your learning agility.

Empower starts with self-coaching to activate neural networks in your brain, which enables you to embrace new ways of thinking, working, learning, and leading. You may not think of yourself as a big wave surfer, but the authors offer clear steps that prepare you to take on greater challenges, and allow you to continue to unfold your mental and physical potential as you live a happier and more successful life.

— Pat Reed, Agile executive, coach and transformational leader,
   Adjunct at the University of California, Berkeley

INTRODUCTION

What would it take for you to be your best possible self—to be healthier, happier, and more successful in your personal relationships, your career, in every part of your life? How can you function at your highest level and make good choices? For a businessperson this may mean making progressive changes that allow you to rise to a higher level of leadership. For a spouse or partner this might mean becoming more sensitive to emotional triggers so that you can create an improved relationship. For a coach this would allow you to understand yourself and the person you are coaching on a deeper level and produce better outcomes.

Self Empower helps you shorten the learning curve between you and joyful excellence. The tools you need to use to do this are based on the physiological phenomenon of "neuroadaptability"— the capacity of your nervous system to adapt rapidly and learn from challenges.

Neuroadaptability is the ultimate tool to Self Empower because it enables you to rewire your brain and accelerate a process of continuous learning. Neuroadaptability is a vital part of Total Brain Coaching or TBC, which is a powerful, holistic system that helps you improve your habits and your life. Self-Coaching is essential to this system because at the end of the day, each of us is our own coach in life and we must take responsibility for our own growth.

In the following diagram we divide the individual self into three main areas, illustrated as a Tree of Life in the diagram below:

- O for Outer Self represents the leaves and fine branches of the tree

- N for Neuro Self represents the woody trunk and main branches

- E for Essential Self represents the roots of the tree

We use the image of a tree because like the roots of a tree, our deepest most essential self is hidden to others and often to ourselves.

The book is divided into 5 parts:

PART 1 ESSENTIAL SELF—Your core values and beliefs

PART 2 NEURO SELF—Your brain and body

PART 3 OUTER SELF—Your habits and behavior

PART 4 PRACTICAL APPLICATIONS

PART 5 RESOURCE MATERIAL

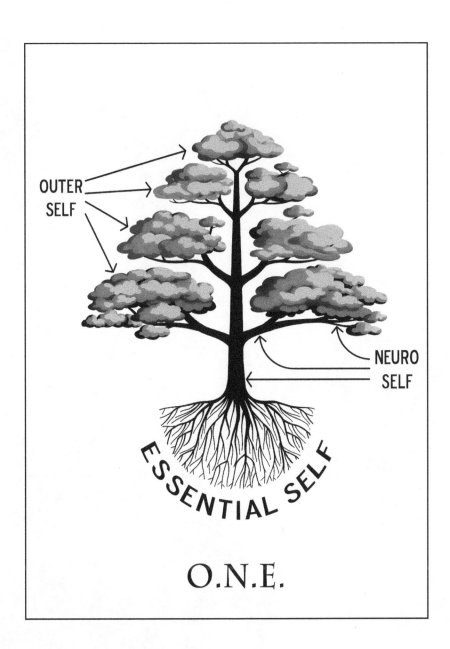

O.N.E.

PART 1

ESSENTIAL SELF

CHAPTER 1

VISION AND VULNERABILITY

Your Essential Self consists of your deepest thoughts, feelings, beliefs, intentions, and core values. And it is your inner Essential Self which motivates and ultimately enables your Outer Self to make changes.

To help you Self Coach, let's look at one of the main tools of Total Brain Coaching expressed in the acronym VALUE. The VALUE tool clarifies the core values and personal intentions that guide your life. Using this tool provides you with an awareness of your strengths and vulnerabilities, which gives you a more comprehensive understanding of yourself—a view from the balcony looking down on the entire dance floor.

Your deepest core values reflect who you essentially are, and what you want to achieve. Governed by your conscious and unconscious psyche, your core values were formed when you were very young. As you mature, they influence your opinions and beliefs, yet each new experience modifies and refines them.

There may be periods when you lose touch with your connection to your core values and beliefs. Stress and other mental and emotional disturbances can create a mental fog and it's as if you forget who you really are. But even a moment of clarity or inspiration can help you rediscover your true self. The key to success is to establish a harmonious, coherent internal state, creating the basis for maximum adaptability. This will enable you to Self Empower and achieve happiness and success.

Vision

The V in VALUE stands for Vision and Vulnerability. You want to create a vision of possibilities for your life and address the important issue of vulnerability. Start by using the Tree of Life to define your core values and intentions. Each of the 7 branches are important to your neuroadaptability, personal purpose, and your sense of place in the world, and are directly connected to both your Vision and Vulnerability.

The branches are labeled to show different areas of life. (See the diagram below.) The leaves represent the activities of your Outer Self and are sustained by nourishing the roots of the tree—your core values.

The questions below will help to connect your outer activities with your inner core values, beliefs, and intentions. There are no right or wrong answers.

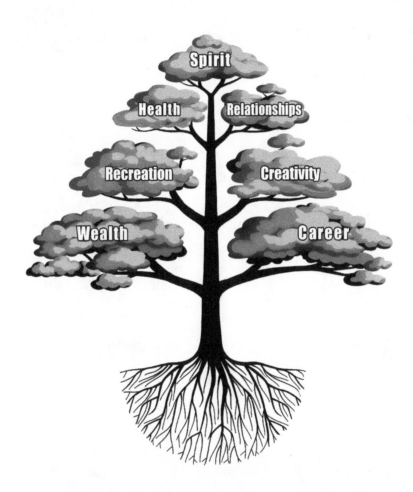

THE TREE OF LIFE

WEALTH Branch

- What level of wealth are you aiming for?

- Do you want a better home or car?

- Does debt weigh you down? Do you have a plan to get out of debt?

CAREER Branch

- Are you happy in your current job or community activities?

- Do you have a long-term plan for your career and retirement?

- Do you think you might be more fulfilled in a different job?

- Would you be comfortable with greater power and fame?

RECREATION Branch

- Do you spend too much time working and not enough on recreation and relaxation?

- What could you do to have more fun and enjoyment in your life?

- Is there a hobby or recreational interest you would like to participate in?

CREATIVITY Branch

- Do you have opportunities to express your creativity?

- Do you have a creative outlet like painting, crafts, writing, gardening, music, or constructing things?

- What would inspire you to put more time and energy into being creative?

HEALTH Branch

- How would you evaluate your average daily energy level? High, medium, low, or mixed?

- How is your mental and emotional health? Do you tend to be happy or depressed? Calm or stressed?

- Do you follow a healthy diet?

- Do you exercise regularly?

RELATIONSHIPS Branch

- Are you committed to a positive long-term relationship with a significant other?

- Do you spend enough time with your partner or family?

- Do you take the time and energy to help people who need it—emotionally, financially, or in other ways?

- Do you participate in any groups or community activities?

SPIRIT Branch

- Do you feel that there is a higher purpose in life?

- Is spirituality an important part of your life?

- Do you feel connected to nature and want to protect the environment?

Summarize your answers to these questions into a one-sentence statement for each area. Here are some examples:

WEALTH Branch

Financial independence and security

CAREER Branch

Rewarding and fulfilling job or community service

RECREATION Branch

Have time for sports, hobbies, entertainment, fun, and relaxation

CREATIVITY Branch

Opportunities to express creativity

HEALTH Branch

Learn new habits that encourage better physical and mental health

RELATIONSHIPS Branch

Have positive personal, family, and community interactions

SPIRIT Branch

Engage in activities and habits that promote personal development and contribute to a better environment and a better world

These 7 areas cover most of the important aspects of life but there could be other value statements you could add. For example, if you are part of a religious or cultural tradition, you may have beliefs you want to include with your core values and intentions. Or you might have recently read a book about positive thinking and want to add the practice of seeing every challenge as an opportunity. So you would add these and any other important core values to your list. After you have finished, take a few moments to imagine what kind of person you would like to be in 10 or 20 years;

consider whether anything more should be included in your list.

Your next step is to prioritize. Life is filled with competing choices. Which is more meaningful to you: your relationships, career, wealth, or spirit? Where do you want to put your attention—on developing a deep relationship or focusing on becoming a multi-millionaire? They need not be mutually exclusive. You will naturally try to find the time, energy, and focus for whatever is most important to you.

Choose your 7 top core values and intentions and decide which 3 are the most important for your life. Why bother doing this? Because there are times when you have to make difficult decisions and it will help to have a clear understanding of your deepest priorities. There may be a few exceptions, for example, if you are a spiritual person you may find that it is hard to completely separate your spiritual core values from the other areas of life.

From Napoleon Hill's *Think and Grow Rich* to Stephen Covey's *The 7 Habits of Highly Effective People*, many best selling books have been written on the importance of having clear intentions of what you want to accomplish in life. You don't have to strain and constantly focus on your values and intentions. Be aware of what they are, let them go, and live your life.

Take George for example. When he was young, he dreamed about becoming a musician. After marrying and having his first child, he had a hard time paying the bills with part-time musician jobs. George had to make some hard decisions quickly. His core values and intentions told him that the well-being of his family was his first priority, and he made the difficult decision of completely changing his career goals and going into business. He had to learn new skills, but over time George grew to like his new work as a business consultant and excelled at it. He also became a popular keynote speaker. He was still performing but in a different way. Now George's kids are grown up and he has more time and money, so he can comfortably re-enliven his pursuit of music. Whatever your circumstances or challenges may be, your core values and a comprehensive vision will help you to navigate life's challenges.

Vulnerability

V also stands for Vulnerability. We live in what is sometimes called a "VUCA" (voo´ ka) world. VUCA is based on the leadership theories of Warren Bennis and Burt Nanus and was first used in 1987. It stands for Volatility, Uncertainty, Complexity, and Ambiguity. Are any of these familiar in your world, especially considering the Covid-19 pandemic?

Dr. Brené Brown is one of the greatest experts on dealing with the challenges of our changing times. Her research shows that in order to be bold and brave you have to be vulnerable. With vulnerability comes the possibility of shame and rejection; what also comes is courage and joy. (See Brené Brown TED Talks.)

To gain greater happiness and success often involves risks that make you vulnerable. This is scary but if you don't take chances and expose yourself, even a little, you will probably spend the rest of your life regretting that you did not enter the arena.

Some people need and even enjoy being pushed to the edge, but such an extreme choice is not for everyone. Many people prefer having a psychological safety net, with specific boundaries that offer a more protective environment in which they can experiment with change.

Being vulnerable is about accepting risk. There are two obvious ways to benefit from a risk. You can either achieve your goal and enjoy success, or you can fail and learn from your mistake. The biggest failures in your life may turn out to be your greatest teachers. People tend to define themselves by their current success, but it is more valuable to be continuously engaged in the development of wisdom and character.

Life is filled with unavoidable vulnerability. Are you able to commit fully to a relationship and say, "I love you"? Are you willing to take a chance in a profession that you really care about and quit your current job? Will you do whatever is necessary to explore a more spiritual life?

The tiniest, most subtle seed of choice is born in your heart and mind, arising from your core values. Many of us have hidden biases which are controlling our desires and shaping our thoughts, actions, and especially our reactions. For instance, if you believe that you have suffered from growing up poor, you might now be driven to be rich. If you were hurt, shamed, or rejected when you were young, it may be very difficult for you to allow yourself to be vulnerable enough to take chances in your life, or fully commit to a relationship.

Knowing more about your personal vulnerabilities, and who you really are, will make it easier for you to improve your habits and behavior.

CHAPTER 2

AWARENESS AND ADAPTABILITY

The A in VALUE stands for Awareness and Adaptability. Socrates is famous for his statement, "Know Thyself," and self-awareness is the goal of many traditions. Greater self-awareness gives you a foundation for adaptability.

To be self-aware you must first have knowledge of your inner and outer self.

Self-Awareness

It is an enormous advantage to be able to recognize and acknowledge your strengths and your weaknesses. Such awareness leads to improved communication with fewer misunderstandings and conflicts. Self-awareness is fundamental to improving relationships.

There are several concepts related to self-awareness and unsurprisingly, they all begin with "self." Self-confidence and self-esteem are significant examples. Are you confident that you can accomplish a given task? Can you get along with people even when they are difficult? Your belief in your abilities is rooted in your self-awareness and influences everything in your life.

> *Once we believe in ourselves, we can risk curiosity, wonder, spontaneous delight, or any experience that reveals the human spirit.*
> – E.E. Cummings

Some people consider it selfish to invest time and resources to become more self-aware. Shouldn't you be at work or with your children, or donating your energy to charity instead of focusing on improving yourself? Self-Coaching is about balancing priorities. Of course, you want to make sure that your important responsibilities are taken care of first. You also understand that you will be able to give more if you are a happier, more knowledgeable, and more whole person. It takes a full cup to overflow.

There is a big difference between focusing on yourself in order to grow and improve, and focusing on yourself in order to gain attention and praise. Self-awareness is a path to becoming a conscious, calm, energetic, and emotionally giving human being. It is virtually the opposite of selfishness or narcissism, a state in which there is a lack of empathy and an excessive need for self-importance.

The Wake-Up Call

Throughout history there are numerous accounts of people who experience huge awakenings, often at desperate moments in their lives. Your wake-up call might not be so dramatic and may manifest in a gradual process.

Motivation is everything—and there are many sources of motivation. Often the fear of who you are becoming acts as an emotional trigger to move you towards positive change. A flash of insight, inspiration, or humility might serve as the stimulus. Maybe you will just wake up one morning and have a clear idea of how you want to change your life. It doesn't matter what initiates the wake-up call. Regardless of your motivation, take advantage of your clarity of mind at this moment and begin to Self Empower.

Self-Awareness Tools

Blind spots and emotional biases, as we mentioned, cloud your judgment. Is it objectively possible to know who you are? In business, different assessment tools are often used to give insight into your personality traits. Two popular evaluations are the DiSC Assessment (which measures dominance, influence, steadiness, and conscientiousness) and the Myers-Briggs Type Indicator (which identifies 16 different types based on such personality indicators such as extroversion, introversion, sensing, intuition, thinking, feeling, judgment, and perception). Other tests are also commonly used, such as Kolbe and StrengthsFinders, and all have some value.

A more recent approach is to consider Emotional Intelligence, which is defined as the ability or aptitude to recognize and regulate emotions and the impulses towards action which they trigger in yourself and others. Self-awareness is a core part of emotional intelligence. When you possess self-awareness, you can improve other factors of emotional intelligence, such as self-regulation, social skills, motivation, and empathy. Empathy is especially important because it has to do with your capacity to understand or feel what another person is experiencing from their point of view. Not only does it broaden your emotional perception, but you learn about yourself in the process.

Total Brain Coaching is unique in that it gives you access to an effective and highly personalized psychophysiological assessment tool to gain greater self-awareness, which is based on the tradition of Ayurveda, the ancient system of health in India. This system of healing was revived by Maharishi Mahesh Yogi, the founder of the Transcendental Meditation technique, who restored the full value of consciousness to Ayurveda.

You can understand your personal mind-body state by taking our Ayurvedic Energy State Quiz. This Quiz reliably evaluates not only your personality but your underlying physiological and psychological state. It also allows you to determine what emotional triggers cause you to become unbalanced. Based on your individual results, Ayurveda offers specific recommendations and guidelines to help you regain and maintain your health. (You can jump ahead to Chapter 8 to take the Quiz.)

THE THREE MAIN ENERGY STATES

The V Energy State, which Ayurveda calls Vata (vah'tah), we simply call "V." Individuals who have a V Energy State are often creative, curious, and enthusiastic. They are your sensitive, artistic friends. In business, they are capable of producing innovative and customer-oriented marketing campaigns.

The P Energy State, which Ayurveda calls Pitta (pit'ah), we call "P." Individuals with a P Energy State are purposeful and dynamic achievers. They may be competitive athletic partners or adversaries. In business, they are frequently goal-oriented leaders of teams and companies.

The K Energy State, which Ayurveda calls Kapha (kah'fah), we call "K." People who have a K Energy State are usually stable, relaxed and good-natured. They can be steady, grounded friends who help you through difficult times. They frequently hold the position of trustworthy administrators in business, and are good at increasing harmony and cooperation.

Current scientific articles demonstrate that these three Energy State types, referred to as *Prakriti* (prah'kri-ty) in Ayurveda are correlated with the expression of a specific set of genes, as well as distinct physiological and biochemical measures. Ayurveda has been described as an early science of epigenetics. Epigenetics refers to the external modification of DNA—turning genes on and off—without changing the basic structure of the DNA. Research has shown that lifestyle changes in diet and digestion, stress management, and environmental factors, which are an integral part of Ayurveda, affect molecular transcriptional and gene expression mechanisms. (For more information, see Resource Materials Section 1.)

Mr. Smith

The Coherence Code and *Trouble in Paradise* are companion books to *Self Empower*. They each tell a coaching story about J.P. Smith, our iconic main character who happens to have a P Energy State. This means that he is a strong fiery, goal-oriented person, who is able to weather almost any storm. Mr. Smith, however, has an Achilles heel. When he goes out of balance, he becomes irritable and angry—in other words, the man has a short fuse and certain situations cause him to explode.

In *The Coherence Code*, Smith's executive coach, Dame Georgina St. George, teaches him that the effect of simply missing a meal, or becoming overheated, makes him susceptible to losing his temper. This is how his brain and gut are wired (along with every other P Energy State individual in the world).

In *Trouble in Paradise* Smith meets a life coach, Chris Trevelyan, who specializes in Total Brain Coaching (TBC), and is highly knowledgeable about Energy States. Chris's main goal is to improve Smith's destructive relationship with his sister-in-law, Seraphim. To do this he must help Smith adopt an important new habit—how to avoid blowing up when his hot buttons are pressed. (A subject that *Trouble in Paradise* deals with in great detail.)

Adaptability

Your basic characteristics are deeply wired within your brain—what we call your Neuro Self. Your brain is influenced by every experience you have, especially those which are emotionally stressful. You naturally learn certain types of adaptive behavior that enable you to deal with environmental threats in order to live through each day. A psychologist might call this "coping behavior." If you didn't get good grades as a kid, failed to be selected on a team, or were spurned by a girl or boy you liked—or if you were abused in any way—you might have built strong walls around your emotions to protect your inner self. Such walls, however, can also inhibit emotional development and result in negative habits, producing future problems, especially in personal relationships.

One of the numerous benefits of self-awareness is making your inner protective "walls" transparent so that you are aware of who you are and what is influencing your behavior. Each person is different in their ability to be self-reflective and deal with inner damage. Self-Coaching is not a substitute for therapy and you may need a trained expert to help you through the minefields. But there are many areas of your Essential Self which you can explore and address.

In order to change your behavior to produce greater happiness and success, you must ultimately rewire your brain so that it operates more coherently. Your goal is to increase your neuroadaptability so that whatever challenge arises, you will be able to deal with it more effectively and more quickly re-establish balance.

CHAPTER 3

LISTEN AND LEARN

The L in VALUE stands for Listen and Learn. Personal coaches recognize that listening is vital to their work. They know that if they comment too quickly or are too eager to give advice, they can miss the deeper issues their client needs to express.

Listen

Listening is also critical for Self-Coaching. In this case, we are talking about a different kind of listening. Self-talk is when you listen to your inner voice, which can be either positive or negative. Self-talk is a topic that many psychologists have written about because it affects how you think and act.

It is a truism that thinking is influenced by emotion. Negativity, criticism, anxiety, worry, and doubt, can damage your self-confidence and set you up for failure. On the other hand, positive self-talk can help you. Your inner critic can become your strongest cheerleader.

How do people change their self-talk? Every year articles

appear about making a New Year's resolution to think positively and improve your self-talk. But let's be honest, your self-talk is a long-established habit and it's going to be hard to change. There are, however, certain things you can do when your self-talk puts you down and tells you, "You're never going to be able to do this," or "You always mess up."

It's important to talk back to your negative voice: "I can do this," or "This is no big deal," or "It's only a small mistake." When you change your self-talk in this way you build a habit of positive self-talk and encouragement. This is part of becoming your own self coach and advocate. It may take a while for this habit to drown out your negative voice. It's like strengthening a muscle: it becomes stronger. with use.

In our book Total Brain Coaching, we refer to an old story about two wolves who are in deadly conflict. One wolf is cruel, negative, and destructive, while the other is brave, compassionate, and altruistic.

Q: Which wolf wins?

A: The wolf you feed and nourish: in other words, what you put your attention on, grows stronger!

If a good part of your life has been influenced by negative self-talk, it will be deeply inscribed in your brain circuits and rewiring will require more of both time and energy. What can you do immediately to support positive self-talk?

CHANGE YOUR PHYSIOLOGY, CHANGE YOUR BRAIN

Learn it, say it, repeat it.

Changing your physiology changes your brain—and affects how you think and feel. If you are trying to be on a positive path but you are being sabotaged by doubts and negative predictions, which is, in fact, a kind of self-bullying, change your physiology. Exercise, meditate, do yoga, eat something healthy and delicious, do something that will alter your physiology—you might have to do all of them! And as soon as you can, shift your attention to positivity. Don't fake it. Pretending or making a mood of positivity is not sustainable and can backfire badly. Change takes time and you have to be patient and kind to yourself, no matter what.

Self-Coaching is the long-term solution to create positive and supportive self-talk and it leads to improved performance and self-acceptance. One type of behavior, which we call a Super Habit, can accelerate this process because a Super Habit helps to automatically change other habits.

Learn

There are many examples of Super Habits. In his book *The Power of Habit*, Charles Duhigg talks about keystone habits, which are essentially the same as Super Habits. His opening story introduces a woman named Lisa who is suffering from several significant life stresses (divorce, unemployment, depression) and goes on a vacation to Egypt. While she is there, she decides to return again, this time to go trekking in the desert. In order to prepare her physiology for greater endurance, Lisa realizes that she needs to stop smoking. Stopping smoking is a significant keystone habit change which sets off a positive chain reaction, resulting in other positive changes that will vastly improve her life.

In his book *Love is Just Damn Good Business*, Steve Farber talks about the importance of love, which he now considers to be a Super Habit. B.J. Fogg introduced what he calls the Maui Habit in his book *Tiny Habits* and recommends that when you get up each day, the moment your feet first touch the ground, you say, "It's going to be a great day."

Daily gratitude is a powerful Super Habit. One suggestion is that before you go to sleep every night, try writing down 3 or 4 things you are grateful for. It's okay if you repeat the same things each night. Another suggestion is to involve your family by asking each person after dinner, "Can you think of anything that made you grateful or happy today?"

We (the authors) recently had the pleasure of speaking with Richard Sheridan, author of the bestselling books *Joy, Inc.* and *Chief Joy Officer* and one of the founders of Menlo Innovations. When we asked if he used Super Habits, Rich told us that two of his most successful business habits were pairing programmers on any given task and then switching the pairs every five days. He explained that this not only improved performance, but created greater understanding and empathy among everyone involved. Even simple habits change your brain and create new pathways. Menlo Innovations is an example of a company that encourages its employees to Self Empower, resulting in greater happiness and profitability.

The Super Habit that we highly recommend is Transcendental Meditation. The authors learned the Transcendental Meditation technique, or TM, separately and have enjoyed radical improvement in our lives, with greater awareness, increased energy, creativity, and happiness.

EEG brain wave measurements and other physiological and biochemical parameters objectively verify the subjective experience of transcending to quieter levels of the mind during TM. Well-controlled clinical trials show that the long-term practice of TM is accompanied by numerous benefits in physical and mental health, especially cardiovascular health. TM naturally creates greater coherence and stability in the internal physiology which leads to greater neuroadaptability in outer activity. For example, research shows that with the practice of TM, subjects recover more quickly from stressful stimuli than controls, and even at rest cortisol levels are lower. (See Resource Material Section 2 for a more complete description of how different kinds of meditation affect your brain and body.)

The habit of being deeply silent and meditating is part of many spiritual and cultural traditions. When you begin to experience quieter levels of the mind, you become open to your inner intelligence and creativity, and as your mind expands your intuition grows.

> *The intuitive mind is a sacred gift and the rational mind is a faithful servant.*
>
> –Einstein

In his 2005 Stanford commencement speech, Steve Jobs credited his intuitive approach as the source of his success. "You have to trust in something," he said. "Your gut, destiny, life, karma, whatever."

Learning always involves the creation of new habits, such as riding a bike or using a computer software program. The sooner you are able to adopt more positive habits, and especially a Super Habit, the sooner you will be able to take action that results in greater enjoyment and success. (PART 3 will take you through a step-by-step process for learning new positive habits.)

CHAPTER 4

UNDERSTAND AND UNIFY

The next letter in our acronym VALUE is U, which stands for Understand and Unify. You want to understand how to integrate your new habit into your daily life.

Change is rarely easy, especially when it comes to relationships. Learning any new habit involves a number of steps (again see PART 3). Continuous feedback is one of the steps and it's a valuable tool to help you understand and evaluate your progress. Another step is assuming full responsibility and owning the change you are trying to adopt, so that it can become integral to your daily routine.

CHAPTER 5

EXPERIMENT AND EVOLVE

The letter E in VALUE stands for Experiment and Evolve. One of the most useful habits in life is the willingness to constantly try something new—to experiment. This is the essence of a growth mind set as opposed to a fixed mindset. In her book, *Mindset: The New Psychology of Success,* Carol Dweck explains that outer growth and progress are based on your inner belief in improvement and self-development. Total Brain Coaching uses Super Habits like TM to help you evolve and improve your neuroadaptability and learning agility. The more adaptive and resilient you become, the better chance you have to not only survive, but to excel in our changing world.

Shaping Our Reality

The advantage of the VALUE tool is that it helps connect you to your core values and beliefs—your Essential Self. By nourishing your Essential Self, you simultaneously strengthen every part of your life. Knowledge and learning are based on the state of your consciousness and self-awareness.

Neuroscience reveals that you are not a passive observer, but rather you are an active participant. Your brain processes sensory information into meaningful personal experience. In other words, you are dynamically involved in the perception and interpretation of the world in which you live—you create your own reality.

PART 2

NEURO SELF

CHAPTER 6

EVERY EXPERIENCE CHANGES YOUR BRAIN

Your Neuro Self represents all the neural circuits and pathways that underlie your behavior and habits. It acts as an interface between your Essential Self and your Outer Self. In our initial Tree of Life diagram, you may remember that the trunk and main branches constitute your Neuro Self.

It is the Neuro Self that enables your mind, heart, thoughts, and feelings, to be expressed as action and behavior. Your Neuro Self also includes your gut-brain axis, a network in which the nervous system, hormonal system, immune system, gut or enteric nervous system, and gut microbiome, are integrated. The gut microbiome consists of trillions of "friendly bacteria" that live in your lower digestive tract and have an enormous impact on both your mental and physical health. Studies show how the composition of the gut microbiome can even affect how we react to stress. In the past, people talked about having a "gut feeling." It is now understood that there is a scientific basis for this feeling. The bidirectional communication between the gut and brain affects everything we do. (See Resource Material Section 3 for more detailed information.)

As we have said and will continue to say, every experience you have changes your brain. The genes you were born with provide the basic architecture of your nervous system, and your early childhood experiences greatly modify the basic neural circuits in your brain. These deep neural networks continue to shape your behavior and habits as an adult.

Your brain is incredibly flexible and active, which accounts for the word neuroplasticity—referring to the brain's ability to change as a result of any life experience. Neuroadaptability is a special type of neuroplasticity that refers to the brain's activity as it adapts over time to experiences which you perceive as challenging or threatening.

To illustrate how neuroadaptability works we will take a look at the brain of our favorite fictional character, Mr. Smith. In one interaction with his fiery sister-in-law, Seraphim, she has set up an actual "honey trap" to lure bears into his golf practice area. After hitting a few balls, Smith notices two fat little bear cubs ambling out of the nearby woods. Moving purposefully towards the spot where his balls have landed, they begin to devour a sticky trove of golden honey. It occurs to him that where there are cubs, there must also be a mother bear. In full fight or flight mode, Smith rapidly exits in the opposite direction.

What kind of neuroadaptive activity is taking place in his brain? As soon as he thinks of the angry mother bear, a small and potent part of his brain called the amygdala becomes activated. The amygdala is the seat of your greatest fears and phobias and is connected to a structure called the hippocampus, which has access to memories and emotions. (See brain diagram below.) These two areas are connected to the higher centers in the prefrontal cortex where information is interpreted. Is there a dangerous snake in front of you or is it a string? Before any action can take place, you normally use logic and reason to decide if a threat is real. In an emergency, however, your brain takes a different path.

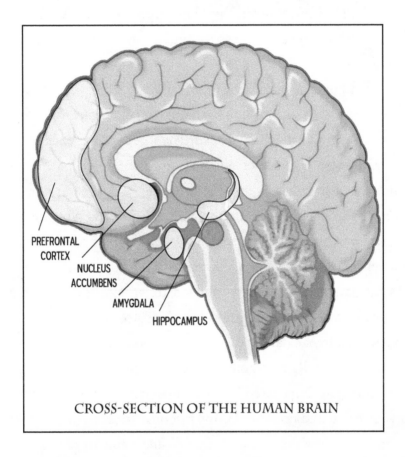

PREFRONTAL CORTEX

NUCLEUS ACCUMBENS

AMYGDALA

HIPPOCAMPUS

CROSS-SECTION OF THE HUMAN BRAIN

Nature has created what neuroscientists call the short path, which allows the amygdala and hippocampus to act immediately, without waiting for prefrontal processing to arrive at a decision.

Smith's brain is on hyperalert and uses this path with his amygdala and hippocampus as the sole interpreters of the perceived threat. Bypassing the prefrontal cortex, urgent threat signals are sent to a number of areas in his brain and body, including the hypothalamus, pituitary gland, and adrenal glands.

Smith's amygdala and hippocampus have wisely chosen flight over fight. His heart is racing, his blood pressure rising, and blood flow is decreasing to his digestive organs and increasing to his muscles to aid his getaway.

If you could look inside Smith's brain at this moment you would see the rise of various hormones and neurotransmitters. For ease of understanding we will color-code these chemicals. You will notice a surge of noradrenalin or norepinephrine, to which we arbitrarily assign the color magenta. A copious flow of magenta throughout his entire body reveals that his sympathetic nervous system is fully stimulated. The release of adrenalin or epinephrine (which we have chosen to color hot pink) from his adrenal glands can be seen in his bloodstream. Cortisol, the stress hormone, is being secreted into his bloodstream by a different part of the adrenal glands. We give it the color turquoise.

The fight or flight response is a huge evolutionary advantage when you are being chased by a wild predator. But what happens to your brain and body when this response is repeatedly turned on in situations which do not require it—like being stuck in a traffic jam, or having to hold the phone as you endlessly wait to speak to a human customer service agent? The result of such apparently harmless situations is a constantly elevated level of cortisol which is actually harmful to both your physical and mental health.

Unremittingly high levels of cortisol can depress your immune system, shut down your digestion, and result in long-term gut problems. Over time, high cortisol levels also have negative effects on parts of your brain. The cells in the prefrontal cortex and hippocampus, for example, become less responsive and/or damaged, while cells in the amygdala become functionally and structurally modified so that they overreact to stress. These changes occur on many levels including the molecular mechanisms that regulate genes, the number of receptors in the neural membranes, and even the shape of nerve cell pathways.

The destruction of cells in the hippocampus is especially debilitating since this area of the brain is critically involved in emotion and memory. You need your hippocampus to be able to compare present and past dangers, and help to dampen the stress response, limiting the secretion of cortisol when there is no actual threat.

Chronic stress eventually causes or exacerbates a number of disorders, such as high blood pressure, irritable bowel syndrome, anxiety, and depression. In the case of high blood pressure, it is as if your internal blood pressure regulator becomes stuck on high, even when the supposed threat no longer exists. Such side-effects are the tip of the stress iceberg.

Poor neuroadaptive behavior can also be seen in drug, alcohol, and other addictions and involves long-term changes which cause genes to be turned on and off by means of complex transcriptional and gene expression mechanisms. The psychological and physiological basis of addiction involves the dopamine reward system.

Dopamine is produced in several parts of your brain, and is involved in different types of behavior, including motivation.

Dopamine (which we will characterize as sky blue) is associated with the anticipation or craving of pleasure, and underlies all addictions from drugs to social media. Every time you drink alcohol, play a video game, post a selfie, or smoke a cigarette, you are feeding your dopamine reward network. Key areas in the center of your brain, such as the nucleus accumbens, will become dominated by sky blue as you feed these habits. But your brain is never fully satisfied—it always craves more. Addiction changes not only the functioning of your neural circuits, but the underlying molecular pathways.

In the past Smith has suffered frequently from Seraphim's verbal and physical attacks and he has developed his own style of neuroadaptability. Even the sound of her name provokes fear, anger, and chaos, and results in a surge of turquoise as cortisol floods his brain. Automatically, certain emotional buttons are pushed which cause him to become overwhelmed by a primal need to retaliate. Is he addicted to this negative response? Can his TBC coach, Chris, alter Smith's neural pathways and stop this bad habit? In *Trouble in Paradise*, Mr. Smith makes some progress, but only time, and the next Smith saga, will tell if he will survive Seraphim's next emotional onslaught.

If Smith is rested and relaxed, he has a completely different brain. A pleasant yellow color pervades, indicating the presence of the neurotransmitter serotonin. Serotonin is the "feel-good" neurotransmitter that indicates a state of balance and rest.

Whenever Smith is praised by his wife Margaret, whom he adores and respects, you might even be able to see small amounts of the hormone oxytocin in his brain—think of it as a nice light green color. The secretion of oxytocin is associated with the experience of comfort and love. While Smith is vigorously canoeing on Lake Paradise, you might even see an occasional spurt of bright orange in his brain. This is caused by the release of endorphins, natural painkillers that are usually produced as the result of a runner's high, or in this case, a canoer's high.

Smith blames Seraphim for initiating the conflict between the two of them and believes that his acts of revenge are completely justified. As long as he in a mode of blame, self-justification, or denial, then learning either does not occur, or happens only at a slow pace. Before Smith can begin to adopt a new, positive habit that will help improve his neuroadaptability, he must first take responsibility for his actions, including potential collateral damage which may affect his wife and beloved niece Chloe.

Your environment will always throw challenges at you, but learning neuroadaptability techniques can help you become more flexible and effective.

> It is not the strongest of the species that survives, not the most intelligent that survives. It is the one that is most adaptable to change.

–Paraphrase of Charles Darwin by Professor Leon Megginson

Your greatest strength as a human being is your ability to adapt and your unique human brain allows you to do this. (For more details on the scientific basis of neuroadaptability see the link to the article *Neuroadaptability and Habits* at the end of the Reference section.)

CHAPTER 7

POSITIVE NEUROADAPTABILITY

We need to be able to react most appropriately to stressful situations, and we also need to return quickly to a healthy normal state. Restful alertness and coherence are the basis of effective positive neuroadaptability.

Drs. Harold Harung and Fred Travis have studied the EEG brain wave signature of individuals functioning at the highest level of performance in business, sports, and music. This EEG signature consists of coherent alpha wave brain waves produced in the frontal areas of the brain. Alpha waves reveal a relaxed state of awareness, and increased coherence indicates greater integration between different parts of the brain. This pattern is also seen in long term practitioners of Transcendental Meditation who have high levels of neuroadaptability.

Most people understand that meditation can counteract the negative effects of stress. No surprise there. More importantly, TM research shows that it is possible to reach an optimal state of brain functioning, with better physical and mental health. There are different types of meditation, and each produces different results. Before you choose a practice it is important for you to carefully evaluate the research. (See Resource Materials Section 2 for details on different meditation techniques and pertinent research.)

Self-Realization

Complete self-realization or enlightenment is a key concept in many ancient traditions, particularly the Vedic tradition of India. We suggest that the experiences of higher awareness and greater presence represent a more refined level of brain integration. It was the great genius of Maharishi Mahesh Yogi to reveal enlightenment as something real and natural, which develops systematically in a continuous and progressive manner on the basis of neurophysiological refinement, utilizing the existing mechanics of human physiology. Enlightenment represents the ultimate development of what most of us consider the most valuable qualities of human life.

For millennia, individuals from many cultures and backgrounds have reported enlightened experiences. Here are two examples from Western culture:

> *The millions are awake enough for physical labor; but only one in a million is awake enough for effective intellectual exertion, only one in a hundred million to a poetic or divine life. To be awake is to be alive. I have never yet met a man who was quite awake. How could I have looked him in the face?*
>
> —Henry David Thoreau, *Walden*

There are moments when one feels free from one's own identification with human limitations and inadequacies. At such moments one imagines that one stands on some spot on a small planet gazing in amazement at a cold, yet profoundly moving beauty of the eternal, the unfathomable. Life and death flow into one and there is neither evolution nor destiny, only Being.

—Albert Einstein

PART 3

OUTER SELF

CHAPTER 8

VALUE AND HABITS

Your Outer Self has to do with your behavior and habits. Habits are motivated by your subjective inner Essential Self, but they manifest through the actions of the Outer Self.

Q: How do you go about changing a habit?

A: You have to make changes not only in your Outer Self (actions and behavior), but also in your Essential Self (feelings and motivation), and Neuro Self (neural circuits and gut-brain axis).

Total Brain Coaching uses two main tools to change a habit. The first is the VALUE tool, which you already have used to create a comprehensive vision and establish your core values. You will use it in a different way in order to adopt a new positive habit.

Let's say that our friend Mr. Smith wants to write a book. He is not a bad writer, but he is having a hard time getting started. He knows that he has to put in the hours and the best time for him is early in the morning when his creative energy is high. The thing is, he is already habituated to an existing routine at that time. Normally what he does is to turn on his computer and start looking at emails, after which he cruises the internet. Sometimes his daily internet excursions are short, and at other times email, news, and social media devour hours. By the time he gets around to writing, his creative juices have dried up.

V

How can Smith (and you) use the VALUE tool to help create a new habit? Start with a Vision (V) of an ideal writing situation. See yourself turning on your computer first thing in the morning, then start to write for one hour nonstop. Imagine what this experience feels like: Is your creativity flowing? Is there a better time for you? Adjust your new habit accordingly. When it's the right time and your writing is speeding along, commit to this vision with a clear intention.

You may remember that the V in VALUE also stands for Vulnerability. (You know how vulnerable you are to the temptations of the internet.) The advantage of using valuable morning time for creative work rather than wandering around the internet has been recognized by well-known experts in habit change. When you begin your day by answering emails, you are using your energy for other people's priorities rather than your own. You are being reactive rather than proactive.

A

The A in VALUE stands for Awareness and Adaptability. Ask yourself:

- Why can I write so easily some days, while other days I revert back to my old habit of diving into emails and surfing the internet?

- Is there a prompt I could use that would help me do my creative work first?

- What's blocking my writing on a deep level?

Assume for a moment that you are a combination of a P Energy State and V Energy State. On one hand, you have a purposeful nature and you are driven to achieve specific goals, such as writing a book. This is your P Energy State in action. On the other hand, you are creative, naturally curious and interested in knowing what's going on, so you want to explore the internet. This is an expression of your V Energy State.

Being aware of your Energy State at any given time will help you understand how to balance and maximize your energy flow.

L

You probably remember that the L in VALUE stands for Listen and Learn. In this case, you need to listen—pay attention to your dominant energy and to your self-talk. Are you really ready to start writing? Or is your curiosity drawing you to the internet?

Now that you know about one of your vulnerabilities, you can take action and begin to learn a new habit that will let you manage your creative energy. (In the next chapter you will discover how to make a Habit Map.) Right now let's jump ahead so that you can adopt what we call a Flex (flexible) Habit.

The first part of the Flex Habit is checking in with yourself and noticing how you feel. Is your V Energy State dominant and you really need some time on the internet before you start writing? If you do, don't feel bad or criticize yourself, just begin writing whenever you can—even if that means tomorrow.

On a day when your P Energy feels strong and you have a little self-discipline, avoid emails and other distractions and go straight to your writing. Practice your Flex Habit for a month and see how it works out.

U

You have now reached the U in VALUE, which represents Understand and Unify. To really understand how you are progressing you need feedback. Keep a simple journal and note the days when you are able to start writing immediately, as well as those times when you need to take 10 minutes or more to first go on the internet. This self-feedback will help you to identify your attention patterns and better utilize your energy.

How do you integrate your new Flex Habit, or any new habit

into your daily routine? You first have to take full responsibility for your behavior and not make excuses. And at the end of each day, ask yourself: Did I do my best to practice my Flex Habit?

E

Moving on to the E in VALUE, which stands for Experiment and Evolve, please note that not every experiment works. You might have to try different approaches, such as using a prompt or trigger—a cup of tea or coffee, a brisk walk, anything that can act as a spark to help jump-start your new habit. Not everyone is a morning person and it may be that there are other times of the day when your energy is high and your mind is clear.

The path to habit change and personal development is different for each Energy State type. Habit change books are generally written by P Energy State people for P Energy State people. Their particular view and experience of life does not help them understand or empathize with V Energy State and K Energy State individuals who do not have the same energy, drive, or will-power. Flex Habits take into account your unique combination of Energy States, and how your dominant Energy State varies with time and circumstances.

Finally, we come to Evolve. To evolve means that you keep growing and experimenting and learning from every success or failure. Self-Coaching is a continual path of self-development and self-empowerment, which serves you for the rest of your life.

Using neuroadaptability tools like a Flex Habit or a Super Habit will greatly help you on your journey.

Let's focus on the DHARMIC tool and find out how to use it for habit change.

CHAPTER 9

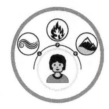

DISCOVER YOUR ENERGY STATE

The word DHARMIC is an acronym for the 7 guiding principles of habit change. If you are not familiar with the meaning of the word dharma, we define it as your ideal path in life. We use the DHARMIC tools to help Mr. Smith adopt a new positive habit of coping with his arch enemy Seraphim.

The first letter, D, stands for Discover your Energy State, and when you take the quiz at the end of this chapter, you will discover your own Energy State. We have already described the characteristics of each of the 3 main Energy States. (To see all of the combinations of the various Energy States, go to Resource Materials Section 1, where you will also find a brief outline of the research on the genetic and physiological basis of the Energy States.)

Mr. Smith, as we have explained, is a classic example of a P

Energy State individual. He has high energy, focus, and a purposeful nature which has allowed him to achieve important life goals. We also know that his sister-in-law pushes his emotional "hot buttons."

Seraphim is also a pure P Energy State type. There are many circumstances in which P Energy State people can get along well, and have fun competing with each other. Not, however, in this case. One of the characteristics of P Energy State people is that they react very strongly when they feel threatened, even in relatively normal situations. Why is Smith so threatened by Seraphim? Did he have a bossy mother who tried to control him? Maybe, but our concern is with the present, not the past.

In *Trouble in Paradise*, hostilities between the two protagonists begin with an innocent, unintentional act on Smith's part. He tries to help his wife prepare a family lunch by washing the salad greens and misses a tiny pebble. As fate would have it, Seraphim bites into it, cracking and losing a front tooth. Assuming the worst on Smith's part, as is her habit, she retaliates the following day when Smith goes for a walk in the woods with his mentor Chris. Seraphim happens to be an expert markswoman and she lies in wait for them, shooting a hornet's nest down to land by their feet. A furious cloud of stinging insects erupts and the two men flee.

As always, when he is attacked by Seraphim, Smith resorts to revenge. The next day when she is out shopping with his wife, he sneaks into her cottage and adds an especially irritating essential oil to her expensive bubble bath. As we have described, Seraphim responds by setting up the honey trap, complete with baby bears.

The battle might have continued had it not been for Chris and Margaret's creative intervention at the end of the book.

The lesson of this part of the story is that it is essential for you to understand your own Energy State, and what the triggers are which cause it to go out of balance. It will then be much easier for you to adopt and maintain new positive habits. So, your first step, if you haven't already done it, is to take the following **Energy State Quiz**.

V ENERGY STATE	*STRONGLY DISAGREE / STRONGLY AGREE*				
1. Light sleeper, difficulty falling asleep	[1]	[2]	[3]	[4]	[5]
2. Irregular appetite	[1]	[2]	[3]	[4]	[5]
3. Learns quickly but forgets quickly	[1]	[2]	[3]	[4]	[5]
4. Easily becomes overstimulated	[1]	[2]	[3]	[4]	[5]
5. Does not tolerate cold weather very well	[1]	[2]	[3]	[4]	[5]
6. A sprinter rather than a marathoner	[1]	[2]	[3]	[4]	[5]
7. Speech is energetic, with frequent changes in topic	[1]	[2]	[3]	[4]	[5]
8. Anxious and worried when under stress	[1]	[2]	[3]	[4]	[5]
V SCORE	*(TOTAL YOUR RESPONSES)*				

P Energy State	*Strongly Disagree / Strongly Agree*				
1. Easily becomes overheated	[1]	[2]	[3]	[4]	[5]
2. Strong reaction when challenged	[1]	[2]	[3]	[4]	[5]
3. Uncomfortable when meals are delayed	[1]	[2]	[3]	[4]	[5]
4. Good at physical activity	[1]	[2]	[3]	[4]	[5]
5. Strong appetite	[1]	[2]	[3]	[4]	[5]
6. Good sleeper but may not need as much sleep as others	[1]	[2]	[3]	[4]	[5]
7. Clear and precise speech	[1]	[2]	[3]	[4]	[5]
8. Becomes irritable and/or angry under stress	[1]	[2]	[3]	[4]	[5]
P Score	*(Total your responses)*				

K ENERGY STATE	STRONGLY DISAGREE / STRONGLY AGREE				
1. Slow eater	[1]	[2]	[3]	[4]	[5]
2. Falls asleep easily but wakes up slowly	[1]	[2]	[3]	[4]	[5]
3. Steady, stable temperament	[1]	[2]	[3]	[4]	[5]
4. Doesn't mind waiting to eat	[1]	[2]	[3]	[4]	[5]
5. Slow to learn but rarely forgets	[1]	[2]	[3]	[4]	[5]
6. Good physical strength and stamina	[1]	[2]	[3]	[4]	[5]
7. Speech may be slow and thoughtful	[1]	[2]	[3]	[4]	[5]
8. Possessive and stubborn under stress	[1]	[2]	[3]	[4]	[5]
K SCORE	(TOTAL YOUR RESPONSES)				

Compare all three scores. Whichever total is higher, V, P, or K, is your primary Energy State. It is common to have two high scores and one lower score. This indicates that you are a combination of two main Energy States, with a minor influence from the third. In some cases, you may have three similar scores. This is somewhat rare and indicates that you are a Tri-Energy State. You may also find that your score highlights only one Energy State. This means that every aspect of your life is strongly influenced by this Energy State.

CHAPTER 10

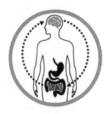

CREATING A HABIT MAP AND PLAN

The H in DHARMIC stands for Habit Map and Plan. In *Total Brain Coaching* we talked about habits as neural networks, highways along which information flows. In that book the H in DHARMIC stood for something different: Harness Your Neuroplasticity and Gut-Brain Axis. We have spoken briefly about neuroplasticity and the gut-brain axis and you will find more information in Resource Materials Section 3.

The practical application of the H principle is to make a plan to adopt a new habit.

THE ABC'S OF A HABIT MAP AND PLAN

A. In the center of a blank piece of paper or on your computer screen write your main intention or desire for habit change.

B. Around this, like spokes radiating from the hub of a wheel, list some action steps that you think will help accomplish your change.

C. Now, prioritize your ideas and focus on whichever action step is most important.

Example of a Habit Map

1. Start with a Clear Intention such as, "I want to lose 15 pounds over three months," and at the center of your Habit Map, write: Lose 15 pounds.

2. Explore different ways of achieving this goal, and list or draw them as spokes emerging from the center. You might include ideas like—exercise more, eat less, follow a particular diet, eat slower, make lunch your main meal, eat a light dinner, etc.

3. Once your Habit Map is finished, refine it by prioritizing your list and choosing the main approach you want to use in your final Habit Plan.

Smith's New Habit

In *Trouble in Paradise*, how does Chris help Mr. Smith create a new habit to improve his interactions with Seraphim? Any time that Smith's threat network becomes triggered, it blocks access to the frontal areas of his brain and makes him vulnerable to his worst instincts. In this situation, instead of focusing on repairing and improving his relationship with his sister-in-law, he uses his energy and creativity to hit back, further increasing hostilities between them. Smith lives by two mottos: Strike First, and The Best Defense Is A Good Offense.

Once he begins to trust and admire Chris, he agrees to try to adopt a very simple habit to help him deal differently with Seraphim. Improving relationships, as we explained, is one of the hardest and most complex of all habits to change, and Chris wants Smith to begin the process with a technique which is relatively doable.

Most of their time is spent out on the lake together so the Habit Map and Plan cannot be written down. Instead, they have a conversation involving common sense suggestions which are especially useful for a P Energy State person. Chris's recommendations would also be helpful for V and K Energy types.

WHAT CHRIS SAYS TO SMITH:

When Seraphim attacks, do not respond immediately. Take a deep breath and mentally repeat—One one-thousand, Two one-thousand, Three one-thousand, Four one-thousand, Five one-thousand.

This is an old technique which is not always used properly. The important thing is for Smith to not react at that moment, but to be silent and focus on his breathing.

Chris also tells him to simply hold the thought Quiet

Indifference. These words encourage a more balanced inner aware-ness and emotional distance from the overheated situation.

Chris tells him the concept of Damage Control, another tool he can use to deal with an attack from Seraphim. If he can't main-tain a feeling of Quiet Indifference, for example, and is about to explode, he does the next best thing that he can do: in this case, remove himself from his sister-in-law's presence and engage in physical activity or distract himself in any way that will diminish his anger and refocus his energy. It doesn't have to be a won-derfully productive activity, just something that will change his physiology.

- CHANGE YOUR PHYSIOLOGY

- CHANGE YOUR BRAIN

- CHANGE YOUR EMOTIONS

CHAPTER 11

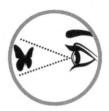

THE POWER OF ATTENTION

The A stands for the Power of Attention. Your ability to act effectively depends on the power of your attention.

Each Energy State displays a different kind of attention. The attention of a V Energy State person can be very precise but tends to move quickly from one topic to another. V Energy State people are more sensitive than other types and can be overwhelmed by sensory information, such as too many choices. Pushing a V individual to learn a new habit may result in a strong reaction. And if their reaction becomes overly emotional and out of balance, it will be almost impossible for them to focus their attention on habit change until they are again balanced and calm.

How does the attention of a P Energy State person affect their learning a new habit? P people are primarily interested in solutions and often make excellent leaders. Time is very important to a P person and they like living by a set timeline, especially when making changes. We have already pointed out that adopting a new habit is relatively easy for P Energy State people.

K Energy people often have a settled mind. But they can be extremely attached to routine. They like to think things through thoroughly and methodically before making decisions. They tend to resist change and will be better able to execute their Habit Plan if they have a little help. This is especially true when they are out of balance and have become stubborn.

Chris describes how different Energy States interact with each other and explains why two P Energy State people, like Smith and Seraphim, are likely to fight, especially when they are both imbalanced. (See Resource Materials Section 5 for a more detailed description of different possible positive and negative interactions between Energy States. Section 6 of the Resource Materials focuses on how these relationships affect parenting and family life.)

General recommendations that apply to all Energy States:

- START YOUR HABIT CHANGE
  WITH BABY STEPS

- CHANGE ONE HABIT AT A TIME

- ADOPT A KEYSTONE OR SUPER HABIT FIRST
  IN ORDER TO MAKE IT EASIER TO ADOPT ALL
  OTHER HABITS

Experts emphasize the importance of starting a habit change

by putting your attention on one simple, doable habit. Ayurveda also places importance on the value of taking small steps. (See Resource Materials Section 4 for more information on habit change programs.)

One useful recommendation is the addition of a new habit to one that already exists. This is called "habit stacking." An individual might have already established the habit of taking walks twice a day. If the person wants to add the simple habit of drinking more water to their daily routine, it will easier if they add the habit of drinking a glass of water after each walk. Does that sound too easy? That's the whole idea!

CHAPTER 12

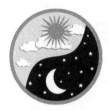

FINDING YOUR INNER RHYTHM

R is for Rhythm, more specifically for finding your own inner rhythm. Each person is unique and has an individual rhythm and speed of doing things. As a result, everybody faces the challenges of habit change differently. Some people are highly disciplined and driven. Others are easy-going and relaxed. Some have a hard time sticking to a habit, others are steadfast.

V Energy Types have a quick rhythm and thrive on variety, so it's hard for them to stick to any one habit or routine even though routines help them stay in balance. V people need the right kind of help in order to remain grounded and focused. If they go off their habit change plan (and they will), a partner, friend, or coach may be necessary to guide and encourage them towards calm positivity, and help them create routines which nourish, please, and support them.

P Energy State people operate at a medium speed but they do everything with an intensity which is very different from that of a V or K person. As we have explained, P people have a strong sense of purpose and are goal oriented. They have no trouble adopting new habits or routines as long as they believe that these will help accomplish their goals. They tend to view habit change as a personal challenge, and therefore enjoyable. If they think that a new habit is not supporting their objectives and ambitions, they will soon abandon it.

For example, a P Energy State individual will be much more enthusiastic about adopting a new exercise program if it is associated with a goal (like running a marathon or doing 50 push-ups twice a day). As a P Energy State person, Smith will naturally be overly ambitious and want to make big changes right away, but he will be more successful if he begins with smaller and more easily attainable goals.

K Energy State people have a slower, steadier inner rhythm than either V or P individuals. They need extra time and encouragement to adjust.

A good rhythm and routine which is suited to your individual Energy State allows you to synchronize with the biorhythms of nature. Ayurveda and other traditional systems of medicine have long understood the significance of biorhythms and their importance to health. This knowledge is now recognized by modern medicine. Simple personalized changes in your daily rhythm and routine can keep you in balance and give you more energy for a significant habit change. (See the Resource Materials Section 7 on lifestyle points regarding sleep, exercise, and diet for each Energy State.)

Regardless of your individual Energy State—V, P, or K—creating a new habit will likely involve some reorganization in your life. Change may involve setbacks, but don't be discouraged. Remember that you have a built-in adaptive capacity and can begin again.

Maybe you are trying to lose weight (our standard example). Eating a lighter dinner could result in waking up hungry in the middle of the night, so it's probably not your best choice.

REGROUP, REORGANIZE, and REBOOT—these three R's are part of your adaptive capacity. Experiment and come up with a different Habit Plan and try, try, try again.

CHAPTER 13

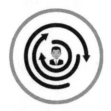

MAINTAIN BALANCE

For Self-Coaching to work you have to stay in balance and M stands for: Maintain Balance As You Self Coach.

Food Is Medicine

An incredibly important factor for staying in balance is food. One of the most revolutionary scientific discoveries of our time is the gut-brain axis and its influence on both physical and mental health. Improving your gut health balances your Energy State, boosts your energy level, strengthens your immune system, and improves your psychology.

In our books *Gut Crisis* and *The Rest And Repair Diet* you will find specific health coaching guidelines and tools to improve your digestion and heal your gut lining. The primary emphasis of this diet is to detox the digestive tract, rekindle digestive power, and reboot your microbiome. It will allow you to personalize your diet and lifestyle according to your individual Energy State which will improve your mental and physical health. (For more about the gut-brain axis, again see Resource Materials Section 3.)

Fatigue Is The Enemy

We can't emphasize enough that FATIGUE IS THE ENEMY. For any habit change to succeed, you have to get enough rest. Give yourself a chance. Rewiring your brain requires energy. Your number one guideline is to maintain a balanced Energy State, and you can't do that unless you are rested. Everything else is secondary.

Types of Coaching

One of the best ways of changing a habit is with coaching, and Total Brain Coaching talks about 4 kinds of coaching: Self-Coaching, Personal Coaching, Group Coaching, and Environmental Coaching.

Our focus here is Self-Coaching. In our previous books we emphasized personal coaching and used Mr. Smith as an example of a "coachee" (this is a real word). Receptivity and trust between the coach and coachee are critical in order for coaching to be a success.

Which comes first, receptivity or trust? It's a bit of a chicken and egg conundrum. Smith's coaching experience with Chris is immediately strengthened when he learns of their shared appreciation and respect for his first two great coaches Linc St. Claire (*Quantum Golf*) and Dame Georgina St. George (*The Coherence Code*).

We may not have the good fortune of finding a personal coach like Chris, and in most cases we must be our own coach. It makes sense to get help from people we respect (it doesn't have to be a coach), and who can act as a "mirror" that allows us to perceive the world from a different perspective. A good spouse or partner often fulfills the role.

Chris's main approach is to work with Smith to co-create a simple new habit that will help him deal with his sister-in-law. Their coaching setting is ideal since Smith receives almost immediate feedback in his challenging encounters with Seraphim. If there were more time, Chris might have asked Smith to keep a journal and record his progress every week. We highly recommend this tool for Self-Coaching. If, for instance, you want to lose weight (that again), keep a record of the different foods you eat at each meal and how they affect you.

As we have said, creating a habit requires energy and clarity. When Smith is overreacting and only intent on revenge, there is no hope of helping him to adopt a new positive habit. Chris understands that Smith's P Energy State is prone to anger, and it is a priority to help cool his mind and body, literally and figuratively.

To regain balance, there are some remarkably simple

neuroadaptability techniques you can use which involve breathing exercises and feeling your own pulse. As often as you like and especially whenever you feel disturbed, you can benefit from a simple technique of Self Pulse assessment as taught in Maharishi AyurVeda, to allow you to determine just how much you are in or out of balance. You can then take steps to regain balance, but the act of Self Pulse assessment itself will contribute to your re-balancing. (See Resource Materials Section 8 to learn more about Self Pulse.)

Your Self-Coaching program can include Group Coaching. This means that if you start a new diet or exercise program, for instance, it's often easier to do it with a group who can support you. It helps to compare notes with others who are also coping with the challenges of a habit change.

Environmental Coaching can also be a part of your Self-Coaching program since it basically involves changing your environment to remove any triggers that may inhibit or prevent the adoption of your new habit. (We talk more about the relationship between Environmental and Self-Coaching in the next chapter.)

Tips for each Energy State

V Energy State

V people generally dislike routines, but a good routine is critical for them to be able to maintain balance.

IMBALANCE IN THE V ENERGY STATE

Causes of V Imbalance

Overstimulation	Too many choices
Overexertion	Negative emotions
Irregular routine	Stressful situations
Cold and/or windy weather	Unpleasant interactions with others
Excessive travel	

Signs of V Imbalance

Hyperactivity	Restless
Easily distracted	High strung
Overly emotional	Forgetful
Anxious	Poor digestion
Nervous	Constipation
Fearful	Irregular appetite
Lonely	Spacey
Quickly changing moods	

Recommendations To Balance V Energy State

Establish and maintain a daily routine	Take extra rest to recharge
Avoid cold, windy weather	Have healthy and delicious snacks
Reduce excessive stimulations	Create a bedtime routine
Guard against fatigue	Enjoy creative activities
Focus on specific goals	

P Energy State

The secret for a P Energy State person to stay in good balance is simply for them to eat the right foods on time, and not become overheated.

IMBALANCE IN THE P ENERGY STATE	
Causes of P Imbalance	
Overheating Not eating on time Not drinking enough water Negative emotions	Overly competitive or aggressive situations Hot spices such as chilies
Signs of P Imbalance	
Irritable Angry Impatient Critical Jealous Hostile Obsessive-compulsive behaviors	Intense hunger Excessive thirst Sensitivity to spicy and/or fried foods, with indigestion and/or heartburn Excessive sweating Temper tantrums
Recommendations To Balance P Energy State	
Eat on time, especially at lunch Prevent overheating Keep well-hydrated Avoid foods with "hot" spices	Enjoy physical activity during the day On hot days turn on air conditioning On mild days keep the windows open

K Energy State

The main strategy for a K person to stay in good balance is to keep physically active and mentally stimulated.

IMBALANCE IN THE K ENERGY STATE	
Causes of K Imbalance	
Too little activity	Exposure to excessively hot, humid weather
Lack of mental stimulation	
Lack of regular exercise	Exposure to cold, damp weather
Overeating	Excessive sleep
Signs of K Imbalance	
Stubborn	Sad
Depressed	Withdrawn
Lethargic	Excess mucus
Lazy	Weight gain
Recommendations To Balance K Energy State	
Keep mentally and physically stimulated	Try not to overeat: light meals are best
Include regular outdoor activity and exercise	Allow extra time for everything

CHAPTER 14

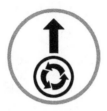

IMPROVEMENT AND INTEGRATION

The I stands for Improvement and Integration, using objective measures to give you feedback. How can you know if you are improving unless you have a way to measure your progress? If your goal is to lose weight, get on a scale occasionally to see how you are doing. If your habit change plan is working, and you see improvements, it is essential to integrate them into your daily routine. On the other hand, if you're not achieving your objectives, consider changing your Habit Plan. Adapt and reboot, reboot, reboot.

Making your environment more habit friendly is the essence of environmental coaching. For example, when you are trying to lose weight, remove fatty and sugary snacks from your home—don't let them in the door! Another thing to avoid is going out to dinner and being tempted to have a big meal. (Avoid temptation at all cost.)

Identify Your Triggers and Apply First Aid

Triggers in your environment might be people, objects, types of food, drugs, or situations which have the ability to set off an emotional bomb inside you. Until you are virtually bomb proof—and you really will get better and better at it—avoid these traps.

Smith's most powerful trigger is Seraphim. Up to now, he has stayed away from Paradise Lake, her home territory, which has worked well. But his wife has insisted on this trip and now he can't avoid her.

Chris gives Smith some simple, effective tips to create and maintain his P Energy State balance while he creates a new habit that will help him manage his emotions if (when) Seraphim attacks. Each time Smith fails, Chris goes over the details of the encounter and tries to help him regain balance and recognize and acknowledge his impulsive and counterproductive response.

THE HOT BUTTON FORMULA

Help Yourself the Way Chris Helped Smith

When Your Hot Buttons Are Pushed

ONE. *Focus only on yourself for the moment.* Be silent, don't say a word, regardless of the provocation. It isn't easy. Do the very best you can.

TWO. The simple habit Chris suggests is to take a deep breath and count to five, which we have already described (One one-thousand, Two one-thousand...).

THREE. Continue To Be Silent and Focus On Your Breathing.

FOUR. *Say Nothing, Do Nothing.* The best that you can do right now is to mentally hold the thought "*Quiet Indifference.*"

FIVE. Do your best to *not react no matter what the other person might say or do.* And remind yourself of the words *Quiet Indifference.* YOU are the person who is important right now—so focus on your breath, your heart, and your body. At any time come back to Quiet Indifference.

SIX. Exit the scene as gracefully as possible without further upsetting the person.

SEVEN. Now is the time to Change Your Physiology, Change Your Brain. Take a walk or a run or do anything else. You might also do diaphragmatic breathing, a popular stress reduction technique. (There are many descriptions on the internet, so ours is brief.)

- Sit or lie comfortably and place one hand on the middle of your upper chest.

- Put your other hand on your belly just below the rib cage. Inhale slowly through your nose and feel your stomach push upward against your hand as air fills your lungs.

- Exhale through your mouth, feeling your abdominal

muscles tighten and your stomach fall in. Throughout the process, your chest should remain relatively still.

- Repeat this for about 5 to 10 minutes until you begin to feel more relaxed. Once you are comfortable with it, you can even do it standing up, without your hands on your chest or belly.

Scientific research shows that one of the effects of diaphragmatic breathing is to lower cortisol levels—indicating a decreased stress response.

EIGHT. Again, experiment. If this doesn't work, reboot and try a different approach.

CHAPTER 15

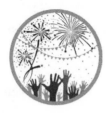

CELEBRATE

The seventh and final principle is: C for Celebrate. Every time you make a positive change, even if it's only a mini-success, reward yourself with some form of suitable celebration. For bigger milestones, celebrate once a week, once a month, or once a year. The act of celebration actually helps to reinforce your new habit, which in turn increases your motivation and self-confidence. Small wins lead to big wins. When you improve one part of your life, inevitably you will want to adopt other positive habits.

Smith's wife, Margaret, uses Seraphim's birthday celebration as an opportunity to resolve the ongoing conflict between her husband and her sister. The meaningful quality of the gift that Smith and Chris give to Seraphim proves essential for creating peace. Giving is an important part of celebrating and it is a powerful tool for promoting harmony and coherence. As your own coach, make sure that you encourage yourself as much or even more than you would someone else if you were their coach!

Researchers at Harvard have examined what motivates employees to produce the greatest creative output. It turns out that the old motivators of fear and pressure don't work nearly as well as happiness and positive support. Big surprise.

Creating Coherence

Greater brain coherence, as we described earlier, is correlated with greater creativity, neuroadaptability, and success in a world of uncertainty and constant change.

The principle of coherence can also be applied to a family or group. You have probably had the experience of walking into a house in which the atmosphere feels "good" or harmonious. There are other homes in which you may feel uncomfortable and tense. There is research which shows that collective consciousness is real and can be improved by introducing certain coherence-creating techniques. (See Resource Materials Section 9 for more information on creating coherence in group consciousness.)

PART 4

PRACTICAL APPLICATIONS

CHAPTER 16

LET'S GET REAL

So, how do you begin your process to Self Empower? We explained that the first step is to use the TBC tool, VALUE, which gives you a comprehensive vision of your life and your core values. The second step is using the DHARMIC tool to help you adopt positive new habits.

Three fictional characters, Vicki, Pedro, and Kameko, each represent one of the three main Energy States (V, P, K). Let's see how they begin TBC Self-Coaching.

VICKI

Vicki is a V Energy State person. A tall thin brunette, Vicki is in her mid-thirties and mostly healthy, although if there is a flu going around, she will be the first among her friends to get it. Vicki enjoys warmth and hates the cold. She works as a graphic designer in Florida.

The First TBC Self-Coaching Tool is VALUE

The first step in VALUE is V for vision and vulnerability. Vicki does the Tree of Life exercise and realizes that her most important core value is Relationships, followed by Creativity and Spirit. She already knows that she is vulnerable when it comes to emotions.

The next step in VALUE is A for awareness and adaptability. Vicki is interested in knowing more about herself. She has completed the Energy State Quiz and found that she is a V Energy State type. But she wonders how she can integrate this knowledge into her life. She also likes the idea of learning how to be more adaptable.

The letter L represents listen and learn. Vicki is a quick learner but she can be an impatient listener. When she is stressed, doubts and anxiety flood her self-talk. Vicki is enthusiastic about acquiring a new habit which will allow her to learn more about herself so that she can deal better with stress (see DHARMIC tool below).

The next letter in VALUE is U for understand and unify. Vicki needs to understand how to harmoniously incorporate positive new habits into her daily routine.

The final letter E is for experiment and evolve. She enjoys experimenting and knows that the successful adoption of new habits will give her more self-confidence.

The Second TBC Self-Coaching Tool is DHARMIC

Using the VALUE tool, Vicki has gained a comprehensive vision of her life and identified her three main core values. She is very receptive to making a change and wants to adopt one simple habit to begin the process.

Having completed the D step, which stands for Discover Your

Energy State in DHARMIC, Vicki knows that she is a V Energy State type.

She now moves on to H to create a Habit Map. In the center of her Habit Map Vicki writes: Increased self-knowledge. She wants to learn more about herself and how she interacts with others. Around this main point, she adds a few possible action steps to help her increase her self-knowledge, such as reading books on personal development, journaling, and starting yoga.

Because she likes to write, she chooses the habit of journaling to help her understand more about her thinking and behavior.

[SELF COACH NOTE to Vicki: Include a Super Habit like learning Transcendental Meditation in your Habit Plan. This is the most powerful action you can take to improve all areas of life. It makes everything else easier.]

Vicki's next step is expressed by the letter A for attention. As a V Energy State type, she has a hard time focusing when she is even a little bit out of balance. She decides to make her new habit of journaling easier by creating a routine of doing it first thing in the morning. She knows that if she does it in the evening her mind might become too active before bed.

The good news is that Vicki has chosen a simple habit that is a good fit for her Energy State type. It fulfills the R in DHARMIC, which stands for rhythm. As a V type, Vicki's rhythm tends to be quick and erratic, so any new habit must hold her attention and complement her creativity, which journaling does.

The M in DHARMIC stands for Maintain Balance as you Self Coach. As a V type, Vicki is more sensitive than other types and hopes that the habit of journaling will give her more insight into what triggers cause her to go out of balance. (A positive daily routine will be a great help for her to deal with such triggers.)

The letter I in DHARMIC stands for improve and integrate. It would be ideal if Vicki has a friend or relative who will ask her just once at the end of each day, "Did you do your best to journal today?" This will encourage her to take responsibility for her new habit and help her integrate it into her routine.

The last letter is C, which, we remember, stands for celebrate. After one month of sustained journaling, Vicki decides to treat herself to a 10 ml. bottle of her favorite organic essential oil.

PEDRO

Pedro is a busy businessman. He is P Energy State person, about 5 foot 9, with dark red hair, and is extremely strong and athletic. Pedro loves water sports and has the air conditioner on from April to October. He is ridiculously well organized, and a good provider, but he can also be controlling and irritable.

VALUE

Pedro has a clear vision of where he wants his life to go. He has already done the V (vision) step and created a 30-year plan. His main core values are Career, Wealth, and Relationships—in that order. He considers vulnerability as a potential weakness for his career path.

Pedro hasn't really given much thought to self-awareness but he does care about becoming more adaptable (A in VALUE). He believes that he has listening and learning (L) down pat, since he is good at following instructions and does well in classes and workshops which advance his career.

Pedro knows it's important to understand and unify (U) new business ideas, but the E for experiment and evolve puzzles him. He realizes that experimenting is critical in the ever-changing business environment. But how, he wonders, is he supposed to evolve? The word evokes Darwinian images!

DHARMIC

By taking the Energy State Quiz, Pedro has completed the D in DHARMIC and discovered that he is an almost pure P Energy State type.

The second letter H stands for making a Habit Map and Plan and this appeals to his love of planning. Pedro is highly disciplined so adopting new habits is relatively easy for him. At the center of his Habit Map, he writes: Improve leadership ability. Around this central intention he adds: leadership webinars, read books, mentorship, and executive courses. He considers seeing a personal business coach but decides that he can't spare the cash right now.

Pedro realizes that there are many things that he needs to do, and one of the simplest would be to improve his speaking ability. He's an adequate speaker but if he wants to join upper management, which he does, he must upgrade his ability. He has been told that a good way to do this is by joining a local Toastmasters group and this becomes his Habit Plan.

His next step is attention (A in DHARMIC). Pedro is very good at focusing, and quickly becomes an active participant in the Toastmasters group.

Pedro's rhythm (R) is strong and at times even passionate. If he can put some of that feeling into his speeches, they will be more powerful and effective.

The M in DHARMIC reminds Pedro to Maintain Balance as he Self Coaches. This is challenging for him. Two situations reliably upset his balance and we have mentioned both of them in regard to P Energy State individuals: not eating on time and becoming overheated, physically or mentally. Pedro is a workaholic and often forgets these simple realities. If he is going to be able to stick to his habit plan and become a good speaker, he will have to be more serious about staying in balance.

The letter I stands for improvement and integration. Pedro understands the need for feedback and integrating his new habit into daily life. Since he is highly motivated, he should be able to rapidly improve his speaking ability.

Now we come to C for celebrate. Celebrating makes Pedro uncomfortable and he's going to have to get some help from his wife or a socially adept friend in order to celebrate and reinforce the progress of his habit change. This will happen naturally when he starts giving great speeches at work because his whole team will naturally want to celebrate with him.

KAMEKO

With a stocky build and long lashed, mischievous brown eyes, dark haired Kameko is a gourmet cook. She has been successfully managing a cooking specialty shop for several years and is liked by all her employees. When she returns to her well-organized home after work, she likes to snack in front of the TV. Even on weekends, when her friends are involved in outdoor activities, Kameko prefers to stay inside and cook. Unfortunately, she gains weight easily.

VALUE

Kameko has become increasingly frustrated by her couch potato existence. She hears about TBC Self-Coaching and is excited to use the VALUE tool to create a vision for herself. She finds that she has three main core values: Career, Relationships, and Health. When she considers the V as it relates to vulnerability, Kameko knows where her Achilles heel lies. She hates her body image but she thinks that there is nothing she can do about it.

Kameko wants to know more about herself and has no problem with the A for awareness and adaptability. When it comes to the letter L for listening and learning, she knows she is an odd combination of good listener and slow learner. Once Kameko learns something, however, she never forgets it.

The U for understand and unify is a concept she is comfortable with. It is her nature to make sure that everyone around her is happy and she is already a source of understanding and unity at work.

When Kameko thinks about the E for experiment and evolve, she becomes uncomfortable. Her life is built on stability, not change. Is she stubborn at times? Absolutely, but she sees it as steadiness and reliability, the psychological glue that holds things together.

DHARMIC

Kameko completes the D in DHARMIC and discovers she is a K Energy State person. Kameko enjoys planning, so creating her Habit Map is easy, but actually adopting a new habit requires making change and this is something she dislikes. In the center of her Habit Map she writes the words: Get More Exercise. For some time her doctor has been telling her that she needs to lose weight to improve her health, and she wouldn't mind both looking and feeling better.

She jots down the following ideas: join a gym, take long walks, stop watching so much TV, and start yoga. Sitting on a mat and stretching appeals to her, but the idea of wearing a skin-tight yoga outfit makes her very uncomfortable. Kameko decides to start with something simpler. Her new habit will be to get up and walk for 5 to 10 minutes every couple of hours, no matter what she is doing at work or at home. It isn't much, but at least it seems doable.

A for attention is next, and when Kameko puts her attention on something it gets done. It may not happen right away because she is a slow starter, but it will happen. It occurs to her that if she asks for a little help from her friends, this would help her get started.

This habit is a good fit for Kameko as a K type and will help her mentally and physically. The R in DHARMIC stands for rhythm and K Energy State people really need to be active and get their juices moving so they can take on more opportunities for change.

The M for Maintain Balance as you Self Coach, is critical for Kameko. When she goes out of balance, all of her best qualities decline, even disappear. She can be stubborn, withdrawn, lethargic, and depressed.

The I in DHARMIC is for improve and integrate. This principle is perfect for Kameko because she is comfortable with being accountable and using objective measures. Her plan is to record the number of times she gets up and walks around each day. She will also ask a trusted friend to call every evening and inquire: "Did you do your best to maintain your new habit?"

Kameko is friendly and social so the C for celebrate will be easy and fun for her. She will have no trouble recruiting friends to help celebrate her wins.

CHAPTER 17

BE YOUR OWN COACH

Self-Coaching is the basis of all the other coaching approaches. Whatever progress you gain with a personal coach or a self-development program, the final result must be to Self Empower.

Since every Energy State type is different, let's explore how Vicki, Pedro, and Kameko each manage their Self-Coaching. We will assume that they all adopt the habit of journaling to help them be more aware of their emotional patterns.

Vicki has no problem expressing her feelings about herself and her interactions with others, and really enjoys journaling. It allows her to go deeper and ask questions that help clarify her thoughts and feelings. Does she still have some blind spots? It's hard to be brutally honest with yourself. If Vicki has a serious emotional problem, should she go to a professional? Yes, absolutely, and not just a coach but a therapist. This is true for all Energy State types at all times.

For Pedro, journaling results in a set of logical notes rather than revelations about how he actually feels. He uses it mostly as a planning tool for his goals and daily achievements. It isn't helping him to become aware of his inner emotions and he would benefit from having some help from his wife, a friend, or a professional coach. Like all of us, Pedro needs a "mirror."

How about Kameko? She turns out to be a good writer and journaling helps her better understand her emotional issues. If Kameko goes out of balance, she too would benefit from getting help from friends or a professional coach.

So not only is it okay, it's good to get help from others while you are Self-Coaching. Friends or partners can help you reframe your challenges and let the light in, allowing you to see things differently. This may dramatically shorten the time it takes to adopt a new habit.

Self Empower

Some journeys to Self Empower are unique. The beautiful documentary *My Octopus Teacher* is about Craig Foster, a man suffering from stress and depression, who returns to his childhood coastal retreat near Cape Town, South Africa, where a remarkable relationship helps him slowly heal and re-establish his emotional balance.

Free diving in the turbulent ocean at this remote location gives Craig a measure of peace and becomes his personal Super Habit, connecting him to nature, a core value from childhood.

Attracted to an underwater kelp forest that is protected from the wild surf, Craig interacts with a young octopus and decides to film her. But first he must earn the animal's trust and over her lifespan of about a year, a surprising friendship develops. Daily exploration of this creature's life gradually opens his heart and creates compassion and joy. The experience allows Craig to reach a new level of self-awareness and emotional maturity, leading to a more meaningful connection with his son.

Philosopher and writer Joseph Campbell coined the expression, "Follow your bliss," and each of us must find our own path. The best way to begin Self-Coaching is to start with a Super Habit which can make all your steps forward easier.

Find a Great Teacher

As you begin Self-Coaching you want access to the very best knowledge from the very best thinkers and teachers to help guide and support your path of self-discovery. One expert can give useful advice about diet and lifestyle, another about career, yet another about spirituality. Although many of the greatest teachers are no longer living, their wisdom is available in books. Search for excellence and see what works for you.

Growing and evolving means breaking boundaries and expanding your mind in a way that you may never have imagined. When you increase your neuroadaptability you automatically improve your ability to learn and develop what is called learning agility. Learning agility enables you to better deal with change and also be accountable for your choices. Only you determine the speed of the growth of your consciousness and personal success.

When do you want to become your best self?

We have said that each of us, whether we know it or not, is our own coach. You have already read this book, what is your next step?

ABOUT THE AUTHORS

DR. ROBERT KEITH WALLACE

Dr. Robert Keith Wallace did pioneering research on the Transcendental Meditation technique. His seminal papers—published in *Science*, *American Journal of Physiology*, and *Scientific American*—on a fourth major state of consciousness support a new paradigm of mind-body medicine and total brain development. Dr. Wallace is the founding President of Maharishi International University and has traveled around the world giving lectures at major universities and institutes, and has written and co-authored several books.

He is presently a Trustee of Maharishi International University, and Chairman of the Department of Physiology and Health.

SAMANTHA WALLACE

A former model, Samantha Jones Wallace was featured on the covers of such magazines as *Vogue*, *Cosmopolitan*, *Good Housekeeping*, and *Look*. She is a long-time practitioner of Transcendental Meditation and has a deep understanding of Ayurveda and its relationship to health and well-being. Samantha is a co-author of *Gut Crisis, The Rest And Repair Diet, The Coherence Code, Total Brain Coaching,* and *Trouble In Paradise.*

She is also the co-author of *Quantum Golf* (Editions One and Two) and was an editor of *Dharma Parenting.* Samantha's most recent book is *The Maya of Beauty: A Friendly Introduction to Ayurveda, Essential Oil Skincare, and Makeup for Real People,* co-authored with Robert Keith Wallace, PhD. Happily married for over forty years, the Wallaces have a combined family of four children and six grandchildren.

TED WALLACE

Ted Wallace is currently an Agile Coach at Principal Financial Group. He has completed two Master of Science degrees, one in Computer Science and the other in Physiology, from Maharishi International University. He is a certified Scrum Master Professional (CSM, CSPO, CSP, CTC) and a registered corporate coach (RCC) with thousands of hours of coaching sessions.

ACKNOWLEDGMENTS

Our deep appreciation goes to our very talented friends—George Foster for his outstanding cover design and Everett Day for his creative graphics.

Special thanks to Warren Blank, Huy Nguyen, and Rick Nakata for their extremely valuable suggestions.

We would also like to thank Fran Clark for proofreading.

PART 5

RESOURCE MATERIAL

SECTION 1

ENERGY STATE CHARACTERISTICS

V ENERGY STATE

V Energy State individuals are bright, good at creating new ideas and projects, and able to learn quickly. If, however, they become imbalanced, they may easily lose their energy and can become fatigued and oversensitive. They may also experience mood swings, and they will then have difficulty in following a project through to the end. The secret for a V person to maintain balance is to follow a good routine. Certain simple dietary and lifestyle changes will also greatly help to rebalance and sustain a V Energy State person.

The appetite of a V person tends to be irregular and their digestive power is strong at one time and weak at another. Everyone likes to snack, but a V benefits from eating several small but nutritious meals throughout the day, rather than three "solids." It is especially important for a V to eat in a quiet environment, away from distractions and stress. When their gut is balanced, the V digestion is quite good. When the V gut is out of balance, the individual may experience symptoms such as indigestion, gas, and constipation.

See *The Rest And Repair Diet: Heal Your Gut, Improve Your Physical and Mental Health, and Lose Weight* for details about specific dietary recommendations for your Energy State.

V individuals enjoy exercise that involves moving quickly and/or gracefully, but their physiology is not suited for endurance sports. They are sprinters rather than marathoners and must be very careful to not get overtired. Activities like dancing, paddleboarding, yoga—anything that keeps them moving easily—is excellent for a V. They do well with a gentle-to-moderate, grounding, warming workout.

V Energy State people frequently have a hard time going to sleep and are very susceptible to insomnia. They need to understand that they must avoid excessive stimulation before bedtime and take real steps to wind down and relax, such as having a warm bath, listening to peaceful music, and using calming aromatherapy.

P ENERGY STATE

P Energy State individuals tend to be well-organized and purposeful. They often possess good energy and a strong and penetrating intellect, and can be good leaders. It is no coincidence that businesspeople and athletes are frequently P individuals. When a P is imbalanced, they may have trouble controlling their anger, or, at the very least, irritation, from time to time. They can also be impatient, difficult to interact with, and controlling. The key to a P keeping in good balance is for them to eat on time and not become overheated. It's that simple!

The defining characteristic of the P Energy State is a strong digestive fire. The digestive power of all Energy States is strongest at noon, and it is best for all of them to eat their largest and heaviest meal at this time. But the P gut is programmed to produce an especially powerful appetite, so it's necessary for them to eat a good amount, on time, every day, or they will experience physical discomfort, and quite possibly, emotional turmoil or anger. When the P gut is balanced, digestion is highly efficient; but when it is out of balance, the person can experience hyperacidity and indigestion.

P Energy State individuals are usually highly competitive, and they don't hold back. Possessing stamina and strength, they are often drawn to organized sports. They are also goal-oriented and often overdo exercise, paying the consequences later. Above all, P people need to avoid becoming overheated. Active water sports like swimming, surfing, and canoeing are all good for them. If you see somebody out parasailing, that person will almost certainly prove to be a P Energy State type.

A P Energy State person tends to go to sleep quickly. But when the P person goes out of balance, he or she can experience difficulty sleeping.

K ENERGY STATE

K Energy State people tend to be steady and take some time to carefully consider any decision. They are not easily upset, and are often easygoing and agreeable. If they go out of balance, however, they can become stubborn and may seem to lack ambition. The key to keeping a K person in good balance is to keep them physically active and mentally stimulated.

K Energy State individuals have a good steady, digestion, and it doesn't bother them to miss an occasional meal. The K Energy State person loves food, but because they have a slower metabolism, they will gain weight easily, and must be careful to eat only moderate amounts.

K individuals generally have good endurance and strength, and regular active physical exercise is necessary to keep them from becoming overweight and lethargic (i.e. couch potatoes). Running, jogging, and energetic gym workouts are all very beneficial.

K Energy State individuals almost never have trouble falling asleep, but they often have a hard time getting up in the morning.

VP or PV ENERGY STATES

A VP Energy State person is similar to a PV Energy State, but in written form, whichever Energy State is listed first is the one that predominates. A VP person is quick, inspiring, and full of new ideas, but at the same time is also focused and ready to complete the project. VPs can be both energetic and sensitive. One part of them is in motion, while the other is steadily goal-oriented.

When VPs are in good balance, they draw energy from their P qualities. When they are out of balance, their V qualities can cause them to become over-stimulated and quickly exhausted. This duality produces a reasonably strong but variable energy.

The digestion of a VP is like their energy, good but variable, and their appetite is similar. Because their gut is partially V, they may be a discriminating eater with strong preferences, and can be hungry one minute and not interested in food the next. But because their gut is also partially P, they need ample meals to sustain physical and mental activity. The presence of P indicates that it is especially important for VP individuals to eat on time. As a combination type, they have a more balanced appetite than people with either a pure V or a pure P Energy State.

When VPs are in good balance, they rarely have digestive problems. When out of balance, however, digestive issues can range from weak digestion to hyperacidity.

VP Energy State people are agile and have good energy and strength. They may also tend to be graceful. VP Energy individuals do not have a problem falling asleep unless they are over-stimulated before going to bed.

VK or KV ENERGY STATE

This Energy State is an interesting combination of opposites. The V Energy State is light and airy, while the K Energy State is heavy and earthy. This combination indicates both steadiness and enthusiasm.

When VK is in good balance, the result is good health and physical stamina. When it is out of balance, VK people are prone to frequent colds and respiratory problems. With this particular energy state, it's important to remember that an imbalance of V will always push K out of balance, so V imbalances need to be addressed as soon as possible. VKs don't do well in cold or damp weather and need to stay warm to avoid illness.

The VK combination gives rise to individuals who have a wide range of emotions. They are quick, inspiring, and full of new ideas, but at the same time they are stable, well liked, and methodical. VKs can be both grounded and sensitive. One part of them is in constant airy motion, while the other is steady and grounded.

When out of balance, a VK person tends to be spacey, withdrawn, or even depressed. They may also obsess on issues and become attached and/or anxious. It's especially good for VKs to have enjoyable social outings and to stay rested, as well as energized, in order to balance the best aspects of their mind, body, and emotions.

The digestion of a VK Energy State person is virtually the same as a KV Energy State person. Again, as we mentioned, the energy state listed first indicates which is predominant. VKs are generally strong and steady, and enjoy an occasional snack. The V part of the VK combination makes the person a grazer, with a constantly changing appetite, while their K part makes them love to eat. When they are in good balance, V and K complement each other very well. They enjoy food, but don't gain as much weight as pure K types until later in life.

When out of balance, the VK, KV digestion slows down and they become more sensitive to what they eat.

In regard to exercise, VK Energy State individuals are a mixture of opposites and may be sprinters as well as endurance runners.

VK Energy individuals can fall asleep and stay asleep as long as their V Energy State is balanced.

PK or KP ENERGY STATE

PK Energy State people have the hot, transformative qualities of a P Energy State plus the cool, stable qualities of a K Energy State. If they are unable to stay in balance, however, they can boil over. PKs are generally large and strong and do well in sports. Many professional athletes are PK. They might not be the stars of the team, but they have the constitution to be very good players.

A PK tends to be strong, sturdy, content, and easygoing. Their high energy drive is steadied by their calm, easygoing nature. Imbalances can cause impatience, anger, and lethargy. They may also become argumentative, stubborn, and withdrawn. It's very important for a PK particularly to maintain healthy family relationships and friendships in order to stay in good balance.

In the heat of the moment a PK might not think problems through completely. And if decisions backfire, they may be prone to useless regret. A PK individual will be happier and healthier spending more time listening and less time making assumptions and running scenarios in their head.

The PK digestion and appetite is virtually the same as KP. In both cases, each of the combined energy states is strong, but P will predominate. People with a P gut have a good appetite, and strong digestion. If they have a PK gut, they will have an even stronger appetite. PKs like to eat, and generally digest easily. Because their gut is part K, however, their metabolism slows down at times and they may have a hard time digesting greasy foods. It's easy for PKs to gain a few extra pounds, but they can usually lose them without great effort.

When PKs are in good balance, they rarely have digestive problems. When out of balance, however, they must be aware of slower digestion and hyperacidity.

PKs need to exercise daily. They have excellent stamina in activity, but must remember not to get overheated. The PK or KP individual generally falls asleep easily and gets a good sound sleep.

VPK ENERGY STATE or "TRI-ENERGY STATE"

This is a relatively rare mixture of the three types and, when it is in balance, shows the best qualities of each. VPKs are often creative, motivated, steady, and good-natured. When they are in good balance, they tend to be in tune with their body and emotions and may be intuitive. Physically strong with a moderate build, VPKs are usually in good health. They avoid most seasonal illnesses and experience only mild to moderate symptoms during each season (e.g. dry skin in the winter, some lethargy in the spring, and mild heat intolerance in the summer).

Life for a VPK becomes complicated when one or more of their three Energy States goes out of balance and it is helpful for them to learn to "check in" with themselves and be alert to when something doesn't feel right. The best advice for VPKs is to treat any imbalances in the following order:

- Start by balancing V

- Go on to balance P

- Finally address K

Keep in mind that it takes a VPK Energy State person longer to come back into balance than the other Energy State combinations.

The digestion and appetite of a VPK Energy State person should be good since they have a stronger digestion than others. They can eat almost any kind of food and rarely experience excessive hunger or thirst. However, because their symptoms are usually mild and somewhat veiled, it is hard to pinpoint how and when they go out of balance, so it's especially valuable for them to learn to listen to their body and use Self Pulse as a reliable indicator of their state of balance.

Possessing all three characteristics, they are capable of different types of exercise. The main thing is to not overdo it. Because of their K Energy State, sleep is their friend. If they do go out of balance, it is usually the V Energy State which causes a sleep problem.

ENERGY STATE CONCLUSION

No single Energy State is better than another and each of us can rise to our full potential by staying in balance and achieving maximum levels of energy, performance, and success. For recommendations about specific Energy State diets, including teas, spice mixes, and recipes, see The Rest and Repair Diet: Heal Your Gut, Improve Your Physical and Mental Health, and Lose Weight, and visit docgut.com.

SCIENTIFIC RESEARCH ON AYURVEDA AND ENERGY STATES

Recent studies have shown that there is a scientific basis to Ayurveda and its evaluation of each person's Energy State or Prakriti. There is a whole new field emerging called Ayurgenomics. Genetic research, for example, has shown that the Vata (V Energy State), Pitta (P Energy State), and Kapha (K Energy State) Prakriti each expresses a different set of genes. See scientific references 1 and 2 in the list below.

Genes in the immune response pathways, for example, were turned on or up-regulated in extreme Pittas. In Vatas, genes related to cell cycles were turned on. In Kaphas it was found that genes in the immune signaling pathways were turned on. Inflammatory genes were up-regulated in Vatas, whereas up-regulation of oxidative stress pathway genes was observed in Pittas and Kaphas. See reference number 3 below. CD25 (activated B cells) and CD56 (natural killer cells) were higher in Kaphas. CYP2C19 genotypes, a family of genes that help in detoxification and metabolism of certain drugs, were turned off or down-regulated in Kapha types and turned on in Pitta types. See references 4 and 5 below.

Extreme Vata, Pitta, and Kapha individuals also have significant differences in specific physiological measurements. Again, see references 1 and 2 below. Triglycerides, total cholesterol, high low-density lipoprotein (LDL), and low high-density lipoprotein (HDL) concentrations—all common risk factors for cardiovascular disease—were reported to be higher in Kaphas compared to Vatas. Hemoglobin and red blood cell count were higher in Pittas compared to others. Serum prolactin was higher in Vata individuals. See reference 2 below. High levels of triglyceride, VLDL and LDL levels and lower levels of HDL cholesterol distinguish Kaphas from others. See reference 6 below.

Adenosine diphosphate-induced maximal platelet aggregation was the highest among Vata/Pitta types. See reference 7 below. In diabetic patients, there were significant decreases in systolic blood pressure in Vata/Pitta, Pitta/Kapha, and Vata/Kapha types after walking (isotonic exercise). The Vata/Pitta types also showed significant decreases in mean diastolic blood pressure. See reference 8 below. In terms of biochemistry, Kaphas had elevated digoxin levels, increased free radical production, and reduced scavenging, increased tryptophan catabolites and reduced tyrosine catabolites, increased glycoconjugate levels, and increased cholesterol. Pittas showed the opposite biochemical patterns. Vatas showed normal biochemical patterns. See reference 9 below.

A study of basic cardiovascular responses reported that heart rate variability and arterial blood pressure during specific postural changes, exercise, and cold pressor test did not vary with constitutional type. See reference 10 below. A more recent paper measuring cold pressor test, standing-to-lying ratio, and pupillary responses in light and dark reported that Kapha types have higher parasympathetic activity and lower sympathetic activity in terms of cardiovascular reactivity as compared to Pitta or Vata types. See reference 11 below.

A recent study also showed that predominantly Vata, Pitta, or Kapha people had a different composition of bacteria in their microbiome. See reference 12 and 13 below. Sharma and Wallace in an article entitled *Ayurveda and Epigenetics* (reference 14) have shown how the time-tested lifestyle recommendations of Ayurveda act as epigenetic regulators to create balance in the physiology. Finally, Travis and Wallace have reviewed many of these findings, and created a neurophysiological model of Vata, Pitta, and Kapha based on the functioning of different neural networks. See reference 15 below.

REFERENCES

1. Dey S, Pahwa P. Prakriti and its associations with metabolism, chronic diseases, and genotypes: Possibilities of new born screening and a lifetime of personalized prevention. *J Ayurveda Integr Med* 2014;5:15-24.

2. Wallace, R.K. Ayurgenomics and Modern Medicine. Medicina 2020, 56, 661.

3. Juyal RC, Negi S, Wakhode P, Bhat S, Bhat B, Thelma BK. Potential of ayurgenomics approach in complex trait research: Leads from a pilot study on rheumatoid arthritis. *PLoS One.* 2012;7:e45752.

4. Ghodke Y, Joshi K, Patwardhan B. Traditional medicine to modern pharmacogenomics: Ayurveda Prakriti type and CYP2C19 gene polymorphism associated with the metabolic variability. *Evid Based Complement Alternat Med* 2011;2011:249528.

5. Aggarwal S, Negi S, Jha P, Singh PK, Stobdan T, Pasha MA. Indian genome variation consortium. EGLN1 involvement in high-altitude adaptation revealed through genetic analysis of extreme constitution types defined in Ayurveda. *Proc Natl Acad Sci* 2010;107:18961-6.

6. Mahalle NP, Kulkarni MV, Pendse NM, Naik SS. Association of constitutional type of Ayurveda with cardiovascular risk factors, inflammatory markers and insulin resistance. *J Ayurveda Integr Med*

2012;3:150-7.

7. Bhalerao S, Deshpande T, Thatte U. Prakriti (Ayurvedic concept of constitution) and variations in Platelet aggregation. *BMC Complement Altern Med* 2012;12:248-56.

8. Tiwari S, Gehlot S, Tiwari SK, Singh G. Effect of walking (aerobic isotonic exercise) on physiological variants with special reference to Prameha (diabetes mellitus) as per Prakriti. *Ayu* 2012;33:44-9.

9. Kurup RK, Kurup PA. Hypothalamic digoxin, hemispheric chemical dominance, and the tridosha theory. *Int J Neurosci* 2003;113:657-81.

10. Tripathi PK, Patwardhan K, Singh G. The basic cardiovascular responses to postural changes, exercise and cold pressor test: Do they vary in accordance with the dual constitutional types of Ayurveda? *Evid Based Complement Alternat Med* 2011;201:251-9.

11. Rapolu SB, Kumar M, Singh G, Patwardhan K. Physiological variations in the autonomic responses may be related to the constitutional types defined in Ayurveda. *J Humanitas Med* 2015;5:e7.

12. Chauhan NS, Pandey R, Mondal AK, Gupta S, Verma MK, Jain S, et al. Western Indian Rural Gut Microbial Diversity in Extreme Prakriti Endo-Phenotypes Reveals Signature Microbes. *Front. Microbiol.* 2018; 9:118. doi: 10.3389/fmicb.2018.00118. eCollection 2018.

13. Wallace, RK. The Microbiome in Health and Disease from the Perspective of Modern Medicine and Ayurveda. Medicina 2020; 56, 462.

14. Sharma, H.; Wallace, RK. Ayurveda and Epigenetics. Medicina 2020; 56, 687.

15. Travis, FT, Wallace. RK, Dosha brain-types: A neural model of individual differences. J Ayurveda Integr Med. 2015; 6, 280-85.

SECTION 2

MEDITATION

Everybody knows that meditation helps people deal with stress, but which kind of meditation is best for you? Recent research clearly shows that there are three main categories of meditation procedure, each with different effects on the brain:

- Focused Attention (including Zen, compassion, qigong, and vipassana): gamma (fast) EEG indicates that the brain is concentrated and focused.

- Open Monitoring (including mindfulness and Kriya yoga): theta (slow) EEG indicates that the mind is in a more contemplative state, following its own internal mental processes.

- Automatic self-transcending (including Transcendental Meditation): coherent alpha1 (foundational) EEG indicates that the mind is in a unique state of restful alertness.

The first two types of meditation construct mental tools to help us cope with life. Generally speaking, Focused Attention meditations train the mind to concentrate more closely and for longer periods. Open Monitoring meditations, which include many techniques of mindfulness, help us develop greater awareness of our body (such as our breathing patterns), and cultivate insight into what we are thinking and doing.

Automatic Self-Transcending meditations are fundamentally different because they do not involve thinking about something— rather, they allow the mind to settle down to a very quiet state while becoming more alert. Transcendental Meditation is an automatic Self-Transcending technique (1).

THE TRANSCENDENTAL MEDITATION PROGRAM

The Transcendental Meditation technique is a unique, simple, and effective mental procedure. It takes about twenty minutes, twice each day, sitting comfortably with your eyes closed. It involves no belief or philosophy, no mood or lifestyle. Most people begin the technique for practical reasons, such as a desire for more energy or to decrease tension and anxiety. Over ten million people of all ages, cultures, and religions have learned TM.

TM uses the natural tendency of the mind to spontaneously experience states of greater and greater happiness. The technique involves a real and measurable process of physiological refinement that utilizes the inherent capacity of the nervous system to refine its own functioning and unfold its full potential. During TM practice, your attention is very naturally and spontaneously drawn to quieter, more orderly states of mental activity until all mental activity is transcended, and you are left with no thoughts or sensations, only the experience of pure awareness itself. The result of the regular practice of TM is that your entire nervous system becomes rejuvenated and revitalized, and you become more successful and fulfilled in activity.

Extensive research documents the effectiveness of TM in improving both physical and mental health. TM produces a unique state of restful alertness (2-4) with brain wave patterns that are different from other techniques of meditation (1). The practice of this technique helps every area of life by removing stress from the nervous system. Over 600 studies at more than 200 research institutes and universities have been conducted on the Transcendental Meditation program, and more than 380 of these studies have been published in peer-reviewed journals. [Note to Reader: "Peer-reviewed" means that scientists, whose qualifications and competencies are on a similar level of accomplishment as those of the authors of the study, have evaluated the work. This method is the gold standard of science, employed to maintain the highest standard of quality and credibility.]

The US National Institutes of Health has awarded over $25 million to study the effects of TM on health, particularly on heart disease, the #1 killer in the US. It is particularly interesting to note that researchers who conducted an important study at the Medical College of Wisconsin in Milwaukee reported that the more regularly the patients meditated, the longer was their term of survival (5).

A number of important studies have shown that TM reduces high blood pressure (6). A statement from the American Heart Association concluded:

> The Transcendental Meditation technique is the only meditation practice that has been shown to lower blood pressure.
>
> Because of many negative studies or mixed results and a paucity of available trials, all other meditation techniques (including MBSR) received a 'Class III, no benefit, Level of Evidence C' recommendation. Thus, other meditation techniques are not recommended in clinical practice to lower BP at this time.
>
> Transcendental Meditation practice is recommended for consideration in treatment plans for all individuals with blood pressure > 120/80 mm Hg.
>
> Lower blood pressure through Transcendental Meditation practice is also associated with substantially reduced rates of death, heart attack, and stroke (7).

Research shows that TM practice reduces cholesterol levels (8). Studies also show that meditators exhibit an improved ability to adapt to stressful situations (9,10) and a marked decrease in levels of plasma cortisol, commonly known as the "stress hormone" (11).

Research results in various areas of health document improvements in such conditions as asthma, diabetes, metabolic syndrome, pain, alcohol and drug abuse, and mental health (12-17). In a five-year study on some 2000 individuals, researchers showed that TM meditators used medical and surgical health care services approximately one-half as often as did other insurance users. This study was conducted in cooperation with Blue Cross Blue Shield and controlled for other factors that might affect health care use, such as cost sharing, age, gender, geographic distribution, and profession. The TM subjects also showed a far lower rate of increase in health care utilization with increasing age (18).

In Québec, Canada, researchers compared the changes in physician costs for TM practitioners with those of non-practitioners over a five-year period. This study is particularly reliable because the Canadian government tracked health care costs closely for both meditators and the control group, due to Canada's national health care system. After the first year, the health care costs of the TM group decreased 11%, and after five years, their cumulative cost reduction was 28%. TM patients required fewer referrals, resulting in lower medical expenses for prescription drugs, tests, hospitalization, surgery, and other treatments (19).

Studies have documented how TM can slow and even reverse the aging process. One study showed that long-term TM meditators had a biological age roughly twelve years younger than their non-meditating counterparts (20). Researchers at Harvard University studied the effects of TM on mental health, behavioral flexibility, blood pressure, and longevity, in residents of homes for the elderly. The subjects were randomly assigned either to a no-treatment group or to one of three treatment programs: the TM program, mindfulness training, or a relaxation program. Initially, all three groups were similar on pretest measures and expectancy of benefits, yet after only three months, the TM group showed significant improvements in cognitive functioning and blood pressure compared to the control groups. Reports from the TM subjects, compared to those of the mindfulness or the relaxation subjects, indicated that the TM practitioners felt more absorbed during their practice, and better and more relaxed immediately afterward. Overall, more TM subjects found their practice to be personally valuable than members of either of the control groups (21).

The most striking finding is that TM practice not only reverses age-related declines in overall health, but also directly enhances longevity. All the members of the TM group were still alive three years after the program began, in contrast to about only half of the members of the control groups. Research on the Transcendental Meditation program clearly shows that growing old can be an opportunity for further development (22,23). Scientists have suggested that one of the ways TM may improve health and increase longevity is by changing the expression of specific beneficial genes in our DNA (24,25).

Long-term changes in brain functioning have also been correlated with decreased stress-reactivity and neuroticism, and increased self-development, intelligence, learning ability, and self-actualization (26-30). One important psychological study on TM shows a significant decrease in levels of anxiety in TM practitioners as compared to subjects practicing other relaxation techniques (31). Studies in a variety of work and business settings show significantly increased productivity and efficiency (32,33). A recent study showed marked improvements in veterans with PTSD (34).

TM is learned from a qualified TM teacher, and is taught in 7 steps, usually within a week's time according to your schedule. Most of the steps take 1 to 2 hours (though some are shorter). There is also a brief but important follow-up meeting 10 days after you learn the practice, and then once a month for the first three months after your TM course. All of these meetings are included in the course fee, along with lifelong support for your meditation program, including individual meditation checking, advanced meetings, and other special events.

Although there are a number of advanced TM programs, TM is always the core technique and will continue to benefit your life whether you choose to take an advanced program or not. (For more information on how to start TM, see TM.org.)

SELECTED REFERENCES

1. Travis FT and Shear J. Focused attention, open monitoring and automatic self-transcending: Categories to organize meditations from Vedic, Buddhist and Chinese traditions. *Consciousness and Cognition* 19(4):1110-1118, 2010

2. Wallace RK. Physiological effects of Transcendental Meditation. *Science* 167:1751-1754, 1970

3. Wallace RK, et al. A wakeful hypometabolic physiologic state. *American Journal of Physiology* 221(3): 795-799, 1971

4. Wallace RK. Physiological effects of the Transcendental Meditation technique: A proposed fourth major state of consciousness. Ph.D. thesis. Physiology Department, University of California, Los Angeles, 1970

5. Schneider RH, et al. Stress Reduction in the Secondary Prevention of Cardiovascular Disease: Randomized, Controlled Trial of Transcendental Meditation and Health Education in Blacks. *Circ Cardiovasc Qual Outcomes* 5:750-758, 2012

6. Rainforth MV, et al. Stress reduction programs in patients with elevated blood pressure: a systematic review and meta-analysis. *Current Hypertension Reports* 9:520–528, 2007

7. Brook RD, et al., Beyond Medications and Diet: Alternative Approaches to Lowering Blood Pressure. A Scientific Statement from the American Heart Association. *Hypertension* 61(6):1360-83, 2013

8. Cooper MJ, et al. Transcendental Meditation in the management of hypercholesterolemia. *Journal of Human Stress* 5(4): 24–27, 1979

9. Orme-Johnson DW and Walton KW. All approaches of preventing or reversing effects of stress are not the same. *American Journal of Health Promotion* 12:297-299, 1998

10. Barnes VA, et al. Impact of Transcendental Meditation on cardiovascular function at rest and during acute stress in adolescents with high normal blood pressure. *Journal of Psychosomatic Research* 51: 597-605, 2001

11. Jevning R, et al. Adrenocortical activity during meditation. *Hormonal Behavior* 10(1):54-60, 1978

12. Wilson AF, et al. Transcendental Meditation and asthma. *Respiration* 32:74-80, 1975

13. Paul-Labrador M, et al. Effects of randomized controlled trial of Transcendental Meditation on components of the metabolic syndrome in subjects with coronary heart disease. *Archives of Internal Medicine* 166:1218-1224, 2006

14. Royer A. The role of the Transcendental Meditation technique in promoting smoking cessation: A longitudinal study. *Alcoholism Treatment Quarterly* 11: 219-236, 1994

15. Haratani T, et al. Effects of Transcendental Meditation (TM) on the mental health of industrial workers. *Japanese Journal of Industrial Health* 32: 656, 1990

16. Orme-Johnson DW, et al. Neuroimaging of meditation's effect on brain reactivity to pain. *NeuroReport* 17(12):1359-63, 2006

17. Alexander CN, et al. Treating and preventing alcohol, nicotine, and drug abuse through Transcendental Meditation: A review and statistical meta-analysis. *Alcoholism Treatment Quarterly* 11: 13-87, 1994

18. Orme-Johnson DW, Herron RE. An Innovative Approach to Reducing Medical Care Utilization and Expenditures. *American Journal of Managed Care* 3: 135–144, 1997

19. Herron RE. Can the Transcendental Meditation Program Reduce the Medical Expenditures of Older People? A Longitudinal Cost-Reduction Study in Canada. *Journal of Social Behavior and Personality* 17(1): 415–442, 2005

20. Wallace RK, et al. The effects of the Transcendental Meditation and TM-Sidhi program on the aging process. *International Journal of Neuroscience* 16: 53-58, 1982

21. Alexander CN, et al. Transcendental Meditation, mindfulness, and longevity. *Journal of Personality and Social Psychology* 57: 950-964, 1989

22. Alexander CN, et al. The effects of Transcendental Meditation compared to other methods of relaxation in reducing risk factors, morbidity, and mortality. *Homeostasis* 35: 243-264, 1994

23. Schneider RH, et al. Long-term effects of stress reduction on mortality in persons > 55 years of age with systemic hypertension. *American Journal of Cardiology* 95: 1060-1064, 2005

24. Duraimani S, et al. Effects of Lifestyle Modification on Telomerase Gene Expression in Hypertensive Patients: A Pilot Trial of Stress Reduction and Health Education Programs in African Americans. *PLOS ONE* 10(11): e0142689, 2015

25. Wenuganen S, Walton KG, Katta S, Dalgard CL, Sukumar G, Starr J, Travis FT, Wallace RK, Morehead P, Lonsdorf NK, Srivastava M, Fagan J. Transcriptomics of Long-Term Meditation Practice: Evidence for Prevention or Reversal of Stress Effects Harmful to Health. *Medicina (Kaunas)* 57(3): 218, 2021

26. Chandler HM, et al. Transcendental Meditation and postconventional self-development: A 10-year longitudinal study. *Journal of Social Behavior and Personality* 17(1): 93–121, 2005

27. Cranson RW, et al. Transcendental Meditation and improved performance on intelligence-related measures: A longitudinal study. *Personality and Individual Differences* 12: 1105-1116, 1991

28. So KT, and Orme-Johnson DW. Three randomized experiments on

the longitudinal effects of the Transcendental Meditation technique on cognition. *Intelligence* 29: 419-440, 2001

29. Tjoa A. Increased intelligence and reduced neuroticism through the Transcendental Meditation program. *Gedrag: Tijdschrift voor Psychologie* 3: 167-182, 1975

30. Alexander CN, et al. Transcendental Meditation, self-actualization, and psychological health: A conceptual overview and statistical meta-analysis. *Journal of Social Behavior and Personality* 6: 189-247, 1991

31. Eppley KR, et al. Differential effects of relaxation techniques on trait anxiety: A meta-analysis. *Journal of Clinical Psychology* 45: 957-974, 1989

32. Alexander CN, et al. Effects of the Transcendental Meditation program on stress-reduction, health, and employee development: A prospective study in two occupational settings. *Stress, Anxiety and Coping* 6: 245–262, 1993

33. Harung HS, et al. Peak performance and higher states of consciousness: A study of world-class performers. *Journal of Managerial Psychology* 11(4): 3–23, 1996

34. Nidich S, et al. Non-trauma-focused meditation versus exposure therapy in veterans with post-traumatic stress disorder: a randomised controlled trial. *Lancet Psychiatry* 5(12):975-986, 2018

SECTION 3

GUT-BRAIN AXIS

The gut-brain axis consists of the nervous system, endocrine system, immune system, the special nervous system of the gut called the enteric nervous system, and the gut bacteria—often referred to as the gut microbiome. The composition of your gut bacteria is one of the most important factors for health.

The microbiome consists of all of the microorganisms in your body, and the largest quantity of these microscopic creatures are the 30 trillion bacteria in your gut, which have the ability to influence your brain and other parts of your physiology. Recently published scientific papers suggest that gut bacteria may be involved in numerous diseases from auto-immune disorders to heart disease. There are even studies which show that gut bacteria can influence how stress affects your state of mind, and determines whether you are happy, sad, or depressed. A new category of drugs, called Psychobiotics, consists of probiotics (or friendly bacteria) that can help improve mental health.

Certainly, you already know that it would be better for you to eat a healthier diet, but talking about it and actually doing it are separate realities. And should you follow a Paleo diet or the Mediterranean diet? There are a lot of choices and they often compete with each other. America is in the middle of the Diet Wars, with every doctor and health expert claiming that they have the solution to a healthier, longer life.

In *Gut Crisis* and *The Rest and Repair Diet* we give guidelines and specific tools to help heal your digestion and gut health. The primary emphasis of this diet is to detox and heal the digestive tract and improve your digestion by rebooting the microbiome. Personalizing your diet and lifestyle according to your Energy State will improve your physical and mental health and help you gain energy.

SECTION 4

HABIT CHANGE

There are a number of best-selling books on how to change your habits. Two of the most successful are *The Power of Habit* by Charles Duhigg and *Triggers* by Marshall Goldsmith. *Tiny Habits* by B.J. Fogg and *Atomic Habits* by James Clear are also excellent and both emphasize the importance of starting small, which is also recommended by Ayurveda. So, begin by picking a new habit which will be easy for you. It is also helpful if you add your new habit to one that is already established (habit stacking).

Tiny Habits uses an interesting formula: Behavior = Motivation x Ability x Prompt. Fogg says that the best chance you have of starting and maintaining a new habit is when both your motivation and your ability are high. He gives an example of "Katie," who likes to prepare for the following day by leaving everything neat and orderly in her work environment before going home each day. She has what he calls high motivation and high ability since it takes her less than 3 minutes to do this. She also has a prompt or cue, which is the time, 5 o'clock, every day when she stops her work and gets ready to go home.

Fogg gives an example of Katie having a hard time adopting a new habit of an early morning workout. She is trying to use her phone's alarm as a prompt, but the problem is that as soon as the alarm rings she wants to scroll through her phone and gets caught up in looking at her Facebook posts. By the time she's finished, she has no time left to exercise. With Fogg as her coach, she decided to leave her phone in the kitchen and use an alarm clock by her bed. This kind of practical solution is frequently offered by habit change experts: Change the environment, change the habit. In this case, by removing the phone and creating a new prompt, Katie changed her environment and made it easier for her to start her morning workout program.

Fogg uses what he calls Focus Mapping to help develop a new habit plan. This is similar to our program of creating a Habit Map and Habit Plan. As we have described, you write your main intention in the center of a page, add all your ideas for habit changes around it, prioritize them, and pick the best one. "I want to lose weight," for example, might be the main goal. Around it you add everything from exercising more, to eating less. You add whatever comes to your mind. Then you start to eliminate the less useful ideas and focus on one main habit which seems easy for you to adopt.

One of the most important parts of creating a Habit Plan is to make sure that your intentions are clear. If you have two conflicting intentions competing with each other, it will be harder for you to come up with a successful plan.

What Fogg and other habit change experts are missing from their habit change programs is the ability to know the unique characteristics and tendencies of each individual. Knowing your Energy State gives you an advantage because you can pick choices for habit change that fit your own particular nature. If you are a P Energy State, you know that you can stick to a discipline plan with clear intentions. If you are a V Energy State, you know it can be easy for you to become distracted with a lot of choices, so you might want to ask a P friend to be with you while you make your Habit Map and Plan. And it may be good for either a P or K friend to check in with you each day to help keep you focused. If you are a K Energy State person, you may do well with help from a P Energy State friend to help you start the process.

Another important consideration is that right before you start your habit change plan, make sure your Energy State is in balance. Again, this is a unique feature of Total Brain Coaching. It takes energy to make the change, and if you are in an imbalanced state you won't have that energy or focus. Finally, as part of being in balance, get an evaluation of your gut health. Believe it or not, your diet and digestion affect both your energy level and your state of mind.

SECTION 5

RELATIONSHIP COACHING

TBC Relationship Coaches help their clients become more empathetic and compatible, drop negative habits and form new positive ones. The coach will also encourage realizable goals for a loving and harmonious relationship.

In order to have a meaningful relationship, the client must understand Energy States and how they interact. This will give them the necessary understanding of the common triggers which lead to misunderstandings and blow-ups.

The examples below are illustrations of interactions that may occur between specific Energy State partners.

A TBC coach will learn to be aware of the nature of these interactions and have the tools necessary to improve the relationship.

V Partner / V Partner

When a balanced V Energy State person has a relationship with another balanced V partner, they will probably be very compatible and get great joy from each other's creativity. Since they are both extremely sensitive, however, if one of them goes out of balance, any slight misunderstanding on either side can cause hurt feelings. If both V Energy State partners go out of balance, their life can become an emotional tornado.

ADVICE:

Both V partners need to stay grounded. V Energy State individuals dislike routines, but the right routine will help to stabilize both their emotions and their physiology, and allow them to be their best selves. V people do not do well in cold and wind and should avoid them as much as possible. (At the very least they need to seriously bundle up well in such conditions.) Sipping hot water throughout the day is a simple but powerful way to help balance V Energy and help prevent illness. Daily warm oil self-massage with a balancing V oil will also help. The master tool for inner and outer balance is, of course, meditation.

P Partner / P Partner

Two P Energy State partners equals fire x 2! But this potentially combustible combination works very well when they are both in good balance because they both have a lot of energy and are highly motivated. They also love competition, physical exercise, and challenges.

ADVICE:

It is critically important that neither P partner misses a meal or becomes overheated! If either of them goes out of balance, arguments and a power struggle will surely follow. Both of them need to understand exactly what triggers a P Energy State outburst. Prevention is key.

K Partner / K Partner

K Energy State partners are like two contented teddy bears. Being on time is never an issue because they have the same slow, steady inner rhythm. If either one of them goes out of balance, however, stubbornness and depression may follow, straining the relationship.

ADVICE:

K people need to get out, get energized, and interact socially. This prescription includes a daily dose of active exercise.

If both Ks go out of balance, they may need outside help from a coach or trusted friend.

V Partner / P Partner

This can be an amazing relationship. The P Energy State partner is powerful, highly energetic, and driven. The V Energy State partner is sensitive, responsive, and artistic. The hot, fiery P is complemented by the cool, airy V. But when the P person goes out of balance, internal fires can flare out of control and damage the feelings of the vulnerable V. When they both go out of balance, the relationship may become an emotionally destructive inferno.

ADVICE:
In this relationship especially, both partners have to focus on staying in good balance. Even then, the P partner must be careful not to be too overbearing or controlling.

The V partner has to be careful to stay in balance in order not to become too overly sensitive and reactive.

V Partner / K Partner

This pair of opposites often makes for an ideal relationship. The calm, easygoing nature of the K partner enjoys and balances the volatile, talkative V partner.

When they both are in good balance, their different operating speeds don't matter. If, however, either one of them goes out of balance, their differences can suddenly result in an argument over even small things.

ADVICE:
The V partner is the more sensitive, so the K partner has to help the V stay well rested and on a good routine.

If the K partner goes out of balance, then the V partner will have to use some energy and strength to help the K get back on track. It is much, much easier for both of them to take *preventive* rather than remedial steps to ensure that they stay in balance!

P Partner / K Partner

A P partner in good balance is always motivated towards action and enjoys the challenges of life, while the K partner is calm and capable of handling even the most difficult situations. It is an excellent combination until one of them goes out of balance and the situation falls apart. The P partner will very quickly become intense and controlling, and probably become impatient and angry. The imbalanced K partner is more likely to become withdrawn and stubborn, and difficult to communicate with.

ADVICE:
Some of The P partner's great energy has to be directed towards helping the K partner continue to be active and in good balance.

The natural kindness and steady nature of the K partner must help to make sure that the P partner eats on time and stays cool!

SECTION 6

PARENTAL COACHING

Total Brain or TBC parent coaching is designed to help parents improve their own habits, and teaches them how to help their children to also form good habits. The tools of TBC parent coaching can be found in the book *Dharma Parenting*. The word "dharma" is used in this context to mean a way of living that maintains balance, supports both prosperity and spiritual values, and unfolds the highest path of individual development. The TBC parenting tools make it easier to resolve problems in the deeply rewarding but challenging world of parenthood.

As a TBC parent coach, you will help parents understand why one child learns quickly and forgets quickly, while another learns slowly and forgets slowly; why one child is hyperactive and another slow; why one falls asleep quickly but wakes in the night and another takes hours to fall asleep. Total Brain Coaching gives parents the tools they need to help unfold the full potential of their child's brain and nurture their inherent brilliance and goodness.

The first tool of TBC parent coaching is to determine their children's Energy State and identify factors that can cause it to go out of balance. Of course, it is also important to determine the Energy State of the parent and help them to stay in balance so they can avoid obvious conflicts with their children. The following is adapted from the book *Dharma Parenting*:

THE V or V ENERGY STATE PARENT

As a V Energy State parent, your strengths are your creativity, flexibility, and your lightheartedness. When a problem arises, you can usually figure out several possible solutions to choose from. Your kids love how you sometimes whisk them off on spur-of-the-moment adventures. But V parents don't always have enough stamina for the intense 24/7 focus and resolve that parenting requires. You may find that your V mind is going in a million directions at once, your anxiety is peaking, and your energy level is dropping fast. This is why you, more than any other brain/body or Energy type, need to figure out how you can take a break to settle your wild V physiology down, and generally re-energize and regroup. Maybe you can arrange for everyone in the house to take a period of quiet time, with Vata aromatherapy, soothing music, and comfy cushions to lie around on. And if you have learned Transcendental Meditation, take twenty minutes to do it twice a day, even if you have to wait until everyone else is in bed. TM is your most powerful tool to keep your V balanced so you can be at your best.

THE P or P ENERGY STATE PARENT

As a P Energy State parent, your strengths are your physical energy, warmth, organizational ability, and intelligence. Your lively intellect can stimulate your children's curiosity about the world, and your warm heart and sense of responsibility gives them a sense of love and security. Of all the Energy States, you are certainly the most proactive. Because you are good at (and enjoy) solving problems and planning ahead, you naturally visualize problems before they arise and figure out how to avoid them. But your P focus may be too strong—you can get so caught up in the task at hand that you are unaware of, or may even disregard, the feelings of those around you, or you overlook a family situation that needs your immediate attention, in favor of some interesting professional problem. And if your P Energy State becomes aggravated by overheating, delayed meals, spicy foods, or someone challenging your authority, the extra heat will probably set off explosions.

Of all the types, Ps most need to keep their cool. Do not allow yourself to get hungry or thirsty. You can see that these things aggravate your P child, and of course, they do the same to you. Plan outdoor summer activities in the cool of the morning or evening. If your child's T-ball game or tennis match is at noon, wear a hat, try for a seat in the shade, and keep your bottle of cool water handy. Ice cream or a milkshake afterward is not only a treat but will help cool you down. P Energy State aromatherapy, especially at night, can help. If you think that you might have to deal with a potential confrontation—negotiating with your teenager about prom night, for example—plan to do it only after a good meal when everyone is fed and rested. Offer cool drinks.

THE K or K ENERGY STATE PARENT

As a K Energy State parent, you provide stability, strength, and loving comfort in your children's life. You are the bedrock, the foundation of their world. With your calm steadiness, you can structure and maintain a stable routine that provides a secure framework for their growth. And your stamina helps you ride out the ups and downs of parenting. But if you go beyond your limits of endurance, fatigue can drag that steadiness down into inertia, and your wonderful calmness can degrade to passivity and emotional withdrawal. It is important for you to carve some "off duty" time into your schedule in order for you to regroup and relax. While you would rather opt for watching your favorite movie, remember that K types are usually happier and more nourished when making or moving. Useful projects requiring painstaking work, or crafts such as woodworking or sewing, will satisfy you more than passive entertainment.

K Energy State people have a tendency to become sedentary, so make it a point to keep yourself enlivened. Exercise is very important to keep your sturdy physiology from becoming sluggish and overweight. And if you can exercise as a group activity, that can be more ideal for you. It doesn't have to be aerobics or calisthenics—a wild game of tag, a brisk walk, or shooting hoops can get your family involved. Lighter foods will also help—think fruit instead of cake; tortilla chips and popcorn instead of fries. And you are the one Energy State who does well with tasty, spicy food! Remember that even though K Energy people are hard to get started, they are much more balanced and therefore happier, when they finally get moving. Do whatever you have to do—even trick yourself if necessary to start an exercise program, finish a painting, put an addition on your house, or get going on that upholstery project you've been thinking about—anything which will help keep your K Energy State active and in good balance and help you to be a better parent.

SECTION 7

LIFESTYLE GUIDELINES

DIGESTION

- Food is medicine

- Digestion is critical for every aspect of your health

- Eat your main meal at noon when the digestive power is strongest, according to Ayurveda

- Before, during, and after a meal, AVOID COLD WATER and especially ice because cold liquids reduce the fire of digestion

- Sip small amounts of room temperature or warm water with your meal instead

- Warm water with a squeeze of lemon not only is tasty but will help your digestion

- Always sit when you eat

- Avoid stimulation, such as the TV or telephone, or heated emotional conversations at the table

- Remaining seated for about five minutes after you have finished eating will help your digestion. This sounds strange and may feel peculiar at first, but after a while you will get used to it and see its benefits

- Take enough time to digest one meal before starting the next

- The freshness and purity of food is important. It is better to eat organic food than to ingest toxins, such as manmade pesticides and fertilizers

- Probiotics can be helpful and have been shown to reduce symptoms of IBS

- Discover your own Energy State and learn which foods and spices are best for you according to Ayurveda

- Periodically use *The Rest and Repair Diet* to improve your gut health and reboot your microbiome

DAILY ROUTINE

(A Simple Version)

- Get up early and drink 8 ounces of water. The water shouldn't be cold. You can leave a covered glass of water by your bedside overnight and drink it first thing in the morning

- Reduce stress through the practice of meditation. We recommend the twice-daily practice of the Transcendental Meditation technique

- Exercise according to your Energy State, and practice yoga regularly

- Go to bed well before 10:00 pm and get enough sleep each night

YOGA

Yoga has long been recognized as a method to improve and maintain your body while you are on the path to health, happiness, success, fulfillment, and ultimately enlightenment. Research has shown that yoga postures improve certain psychological conditions, including anxiety and depression, and provide health benefits for those with high blood pressure, various pain syndromes, and immune disorders.

Choose whichever form of yoga best suits your individual nature, age, and needs. We recommend the Maharishi Yoga Asana program because it is especially respectful of your body and consciousness, and supports the experience of transcendence.

THE CYCLES OF LIFE and SUCCESSFUL AGING

According to Ayurveda, there are three main stages of life, which are based on the three doshas (also known as nature or Energy States—Vata, Pitta, and Kapha, or V, P, and K). During the first part of the lives of all children, the Kapha quality predominates regardless of one's individual nature. This is good for growth and gives a sense of contentment and happiness. If the childhood situation isn't very good, the Kapha time of life can often serve as a sort of cushion to help them get through the tough times.

As we grow out of childhood, we enter the middle, Pitta or P, stage of life. This is a more capable and responsible time, when we accomplish bigger things and may start a family.

Finally, at about the age of 60, everyone enters the last and most sensitive Vata or V period of life. Many problems can arise during this period, as a result of getting older and because V is easily imbalanced at this time.

TO LIVE LONGER, Ayurveda recommends 4 Simple Steps:

- Follow the Ayurvedic guidelines for better digestion

- Eat according to your Energy State

- Exercise regularly according to your Energy State

- Follow an Ayurvedic daily routine including Transcendental Meditation

SECTION 8

SELF PULSE

Because your cardiovascular system extends throughout your body, from your eyeballs to your liver to the joints of your big toe, it carries a wealth of information about how your physiology is functioning. Ayurvedic physicians are trained to "read" and decode this information by simply feeling the pulse in your wrist with three fingers. In this way they are able to assess balances and imbalances, and even detect disease. When you learn a simplified method of Self Pulse assessment, you will be able to keep track of the amount of balance or imbalance of your Energy State or States.

Let's start:

- It's very important to note that women always feel the pulse which beats in their left wrist, while men feel the pulse in the right wrist.

- A woman uses the fingertips of her right hand to feel her left wrist.

- A man uses the fingertips of his left hand to feel his right wrist. When we talk about the fingers and the hand, we are referring to a woman's right hand, or a man's left hand.

- The styloid process is a bony projection located about a finger's width below the base of your thumb. Use the index finger of your other hand to feel it sticking out: This is the reference point for placing your fingers.

- To take your own pulse, extend your arm out in front of you—right arm for men, left for women—in a comfortable position, slightly bent at the elbow, with your palm facing up. Now wrap your other hand around your wrist from behind. You are cradling the back of your wrist in the palm of your other hand. Now curl the middle three fingers—index, middle, and ring fingers—over the top of your wrist.

- Position your index finger below the prominent bony bump of the styloid process, so that it's just beside the edge of the rise of this bone.

- Now line up your middle and ring fingers below your index finger so the three are touching each other easily side by side. And make sure the three fingers are completely level; raise your thumb and little finger slightly so they're not touching your wrist. This is the position your fingers will always be in when you take your pulse.

- Continue to slide your three fingers over and down your wrist about a quarter of an inch. Now you are ready to feel your pulse: using your fingertips, very gently press all three fingers down until you can feel the pulse beating along the radial artery. It's important to use all three fingers together and make sure that your three fingertips are approximately level, sitting in a nice line at the same level of the pulse. When you can feel the beat of your pulse in any one, or all, of your fingertips, you will have reached the first stage of pulse reading.

- Each of your three fingers corresponds to one of the three main Energy States: the index finger for V Energy State or Vata; the middle finger for P Energy State or Pitta; the ring finger for K Energy State or Kapha. (Kapha may be so relaxed, or there may be so little Kapha, that it might be hard to feel it at all.)

- Feel the pulse beneath each finger. (It can help to close your eyes.) Which finger feels the strongest pulse? For example, if you feel it most strongly under your middle finger, that indicates that the P Energy State is strong.

- You may or may not feel a pulsation beneath all three fingertips—this is perfectly normal. In fact, most people feel their pulse under one or two fingers; only a few feel it under all three. If you're predominately a V Energy State person, for example, the pulse under your index finger will be strong. You may feel little or nothing under the other two fingers. This doesn't necessarily mean that you are imbalanced—it does means that at this time, your physiology has less P fire or K solidity in it.

- What is the quality of your pulse? If it feels clear and the impulses seem coordinated—if it feels good to you overall—this indicates that your physiology is in good balance. If your pulse feels ragged or disconnected, with some impulses very weak while others are very pronounced, this tells you that you probably want to start getting yourself back in balance.

- For example, you may feel that the P Energy State or Pitta area is pulsating very strongly under your index finger, which indicates that your P Energy State is too strong and has invaded the V Energy State or Vata territory. If this is the case, then it's time to stay cool and eat on time—just not at your favorite spicy Mexican restaurant.

- If the pulse under your ring finger feels quick and irregular, you need to get your V Energy State in better balance. Slow down, stay out of the cold wind, and stick to a regular routine.

- If your K Energy State or Kapha feels very strong and dense under your middle finger, you may find that your digestion is sluggish and your mind is a bit dull. Try to balance your aggravated K Energy State with some physical activity and cut out "heavy" foods such as rich desserts and mashed potatoes.

SECTION 9

GROUP DYNAMICS OF CONSCIOUSNESS

GROUP PRACTICE OF TRANSCENDENTAL
MEDITATION AND MORE ADVANCED TECHNIQUES

The collective consciousness of any company or any group of people is the sum of the consciousness of all of the individuals in that company or group. When the collective consciousness is incoherent, the company will almost certainly lack a clear mission and have many internal problems. When the collective consciousness is coherent, the company will have a unified mission—a clear intention of its purpose—and will demonstrate optimal teamwork and performance.

The concept of a collective consciousness which underlies and influences the structure of society has been expressed by many great thinkers. Some sophisticated sociological theories have vaguely described it as a social field or an interlocking network of social and behavioral interactions within specific economic and environmental conditions.

Maharishi Mahesh Yogi, founder of the Transcendental Meditation technique, was the first to encourage scientific research on the concept of collective consciousness. Many scientific papers, published in peer-reviewed journals, verify the practical application of Maharishi's concepts. Many of the comments about the group dynamics of consciousness can be found in Maharishi's books.

In 1960, Maharishi predicted that one percent of a population practicing the Transcendental Meditation technique would produce measurable improvements in the quality of life for the whole population. This phenomenon was first studied in 1974 and was referred to as the "Maharishi Effect." In 1976, Maharishi brought out several advanced programs derived from the Vedic tradition, which greatly enhanced the Maharishi Effect. Scientists found that when even the square root of one percent of any population practices these programs in a group, there is a measurable marked reduction in violence and an improvement in the quality of life, a type of macroscopic field effect of coherence.

A large number of studies have documented the beneficial effects of the practice of TM and its advanced programs on reducing crime and violence and improving the quality of life in different areas of the world. One demonstration project was conducted in 1993 in Washington, DC by Dr. John Hagelin and colleagues. An independent panel of more than twenty sociologists, criminologists, and members of the Washington, DC government and police department advised on the study design and reviewed the analysis of the findings. The study included over 4000 people gathered in

Washington to participate in a "peace assembly," practicing TM and specific related advanced programs for extended periods. Results showed that as the group size increased, there was a highly significant decrease in violent crime.

A remarkable aspect of this study was that it took place in the summer, when the weather is especially hot in Washington. In fact, the police chief of Washington, who sat on the independent board of researchers monitoring the project, said in an interview, "The only way this group can lower crime by 20 percent in Washington in August is if we have two feet of snow!" In fact, the meditating group lowered crime by 23.6 percent.

How could such a thing happen? The individuals in the group didn't go out on the streets and physically stop people from committing crimes. They simply meditated quietly together in various locations around the city. The coherence effect which they created in the collective consciousness of the city was similar to the result of throwing a pebble in a pond: ripples of higher, more coherent waves of consciousness went out in all directions, creating sufficient coherence in the collective consciousness of the city so that crime was spontaneously reduced.

Research demonstrates that it is possible to influence the collective consciousness of society through the group practice of the TM technique and its advanced programs.

Selected References

Hagelin JS, et al. Effects of group practice of the Transcendental Meditation program on preventing violent crime in Washington, DC: results of the National Demonstration Project, June-July 1993. *Social Indicators Research* 47: 153-201, 1999

Orme-Johnson DW, et al. International peace project in the Middle East: The effect of the Maharishi Technology of the Unified Field. *Journal of Conflict Resolution* 32: 776–812, 1988

Orme-Johnson DW, et al. The long-term effects of the Maharishi Technology of the Unified Field on the quality of life in the United States (1960 to 1983). *Social Science Perspectives Journal* 2:127-146, 1988

Orme-Johnson DW, et al. Preventing terrorism and international conflict: Effects of large assemblies of participants in the Transcendental Meditation and TM-Sidhi programs. *Journal of Offender Rehabilitation* 36: 283–302, 2003

Brown CL. Overcoming barriers to use of promising research among elite Middle East policy groups. *Journal of Social Behavior and Personality* 17:489-546, 2005

Cavanaugh KL. Time series analysis of U.S. and Canadian inflation and unemployment: A test of a field-theoretic hypothesis. *Proceedings of the American Statistical Association, Business and Economics Statistics Section* (Alexandria, VA: American Statistical Association): 799–804, 1987

Cavanaugh KL, King KD. Simultaneous transfer function analysis of Okun's misery index: Improvements in the economic quality of life through Maharishi's Vedic Science and technology of consciousness. *Proceedings of the American Statistical Association, Business and Economics Statistics Section* (Alexandria, VA: American Statistical

Association): 491–496, 1988

Davies JL. Alleviating political violence through enhancing coherence in collective consciousness. *Dissertation Abstracts International* 49(8): 2381A, 1989

Gelderloos P, et al. The dynamics of US–Soviet relations, 1979–1986: Effects of reducing social stress through the Transcendental Meditation and TM-Sidhi program. *Proceedings of the Social Statistics Section of the American Statistical Association* (Alexandria, VA: American Statistical Association): 297–302, 1990

Dillbeck MC. Test of a field theory of consciousness and social change: Time series analysis of participation in the TM-Sidhi program and reduction of violent death in the U.S. *Social Indicators Research* 22: 399–418, 1990

Assimakis PD, Dillbeck MC. Time series analysis of improved quality of life in Canada: Social change, collective consciousness, and the TM-Sidhi program. *Psychological Reports* 76: 1171–1193, 1995

Hatchard GD, et al. A model for social improvement. Time series analysis of a phase transition to reduced crime in Merseyside metropolitan area. *Psychology, Crime, and Law* 2: 165–174, 1996

Dillbeck MC, et al. The Transcendental Meditation program and crime rate change in a sample of forty-eight cities. *Journal of Crime and Justice* 4: 25–45, 1981

Dillbeck MC, et al. Test of a field model of consciousness and social change: The Transcendental Meditation and TM-Sidhi program and decreased urban crime. *The Journal of Mind and Behavior* 9: 457–486, 1988

Dillbeck MC. et al. Consciousness as a field: The Transcendental

Meditation and TM-Sidhi program and changes in social indicators. *The Journal of Mind and Behavior* 8: 67–104, 1987.

SECTION 10

HEALTH COACHING

The current profession of health coaching ranges from helping to support patients in conventional hospitals, to working in an alternative wellness health setting with clients who are more interested in natural and traditional health care.

TBC health coaches use a unique, integrative approach that combines the time-tested knowledge of Ayurveda along with the latest scientific research in modern medicine. A TBC health coach will help clients create positive health habits, while educating them about the most effective personalized preventive programs.

TBC health coaching begins by establishing trust with the client. The coach helps the client identify realistic, healthy goals in areas such as diet, exercise, sleep, and stress management. Everyone is different. Using the Energy State assessment tool helps greatly.

One of the most important new areas in health is the understanding of the gut-brain axis and its impact on all aspects of mental and physical wellbeing. TBC health coaches will provide the latest knowledge and how it relates to each Energy State.

To gain a more profound understanding of Ayurveda and Integrative Medicine, it is ideal for TBC health coaches to take the online Master's degree program in Maharishi AyurVeda and Integrative Medicine at Maharishi International University, in Fairfield, Iowa. One unique feature of this program is advanced training in Ayurveda pulse diagnosis (see Resource Materials Section 8).

MAHARISHI AYURVEDA DEGREE PROGRAMS

Maharishi AyurVeda is a revival of Ayurveda, which includes a profound understand of consciousness and Transcendental Meditation, as well as an advanced methodology of pulse diagnosis. MIU offers an online Master of Science degree in Maharishi AyurVeda and Integrative Medicine. The program is a 3-year part-time online program, which integrates the ancient knowledge of Ayurveda with what has been discovered by modern medicine. It is taught by qualified doctors, and students are given in-residence clinical training by Maharishi AyurVeda experts for two weeks each year. MIU is a member of the National Ayurvedic Medical Association and is accredited by the Higher Learning Commission. MIU also offers an online and in-residence BA in Ayurveda Wellness and Integrative Health. See MIU.edu for more details.

SECTION 11

BEAUTY AND ESSENTIAL OIL SKINCARE

Samantha Wallace and Robert Keith Wallace, PhD, have written *The Maya of Beauty: A Friendly Introduction to Ayurveda, Essential Oil Skincare, and Makeup for Real People.* The book includes a quiz to determine your True Skin Type and explains how understanding your True Skin Type provides you with an extraordinarily personal guide to caring for your skin, your health, and your inner and outer beauty at any age.

It is the authors' intention that after reading this book, you can look at the label of any skincare product and be able to answer three important questions:

- *Does it contain oils that are good for my particular skin?*

- *Are the Essential Oils listed worth the price?*

- *Are there any chemicals I should check for toxicity?*

SECTION 12

DAVID LYNCH FOUNDATION

The David Lynch Foundation for education and world peace is a global charitable foundation founded by film director David Lynch. The Foundation aims to prevent and eradicate trauma and stress among at-risk populations through promoting widespread implementation of the evidence-based Transcendental Meditation program in order to improve their health, cognitive capabilities, and performance in life.

At-risk populations suffer from epidemic levels of chronic stress and stress-related disorders—fueling violence, crime, and soaring health costs, and compromising the effectiveness of education, health, rehabilitation, and vocational programs now in place. Since its founding in 2005, the David Lynch Foundation, a 501(c) (3) organization, has helped to bring the stress-reducing Transcendental Meditation technique to more than 500,000 children and adults around the world. The Foundation focuses on underserved inner-city students; veterans with PTSD and their families; and women and children who are survivors of violence and abuse.

The David Lynch Foundation has organized and hosted scientific and professional conferences on business, education, veterans, corrections, and rehabilitation as well as "town hall" meetings to educate leaders and the general public about the benefits of Transcendental Meditation. In addition, the Foundation funds university and medical school research to assess the effects of the program on academic performance, ADHD and other learning disorders, anxiety, depression, substance abuse, cardiovascular disease, post-traumatic stress disorder, and diabetes.

The Foundation has worked with other private foundations and government agencies, including the National Institutes of Health, General Motors Foundation, the Chrysler Foundation, the Kellogg Foundation, the American Indian Education Association, and Indian Health Services, along with numerous school districts and state departments of corrections.

[Note to Reader: The TM program has been endorsed and supported by a number of well-known individuals including Tom Hanks, Martin Scorsese, Ellen DeGeneres, Jerry Seinfeld, Paul McCartney, George Stephanopoulos, Katy Perry, and Hugh Jackman, among many others.]

REFERENCES

USEFUL WEBSITES

Totalbraincoaching.com

TM.org

MIU.edu

Coherenceeffect.com

USEFUL BOOKS

Coaching

Total Brain Coaching: A Holistic System of Effective Habit Change For the Individual, Team, and Organization by Ted Wallace, MS, Robert Keith Wallace, PhD, and Samantha Wallace, Dharma Publications, 2020

The Smith Saga

Trouble in Paradise—A Humorous Story: Change Your Habits In 7 Steps with Total Brain Coaching by Robert Keith Wallace, PhD, Samantha Wallace, Ted Wallace, MS, Dharma Publications, 2020

Quantum Golf: The Path to Golf Mastery New and Revised Second

Editions by Kjell Enhager, Robert Keith Wallace,PhD, Samantha Wallace, Dharma Publications, 2021, in press

The Coherence Code: How to Maximize Your Performance And Success in Business—For Individuals, Teams, and Organizations by Robert Keith Wallace, PhD, Ted Wallace, MS, Samantha Wallace, Dharma Publications, 2020

The Maya of Beauty: A Friendly Introduction to Ayurveda, Essential Oil Skincare, and Makeup for Real People by Samantha Wallace and Robert Keith Wallace, PhD, Dharma Publications, in press

Habit Change

Tiny Habits: The Small Changes That Change Everything by BJ Fogg, Houghton Mifflin Harcourt, 2019

The Power of Habit: Why We Do What We Do in Life and Business by Charles Duhigg, Random House, 2012

Atomic Habits: An Easy & Proven Way to Build Good Habits & Break Bad Ones by James Clear, Avery, 2018

Triggers: Creating Behavior That Lasts—Becoming the Person You Want to Be by Marshall Goldsmith and Mark Reiter, Crown Business, 2015

Chatter: The Voice in Our Head, Why It Matters, and How to Harness It by Ethan Kross, Crown, 2021

Balancing Your Energy State

Gut Crisis: How Diet, Probiotics, and Friendly Bacteria Help You Lose Weight and Heal Your Body and Mind by Robert Keith Wallace, PhD, and Samantha Wallace, Dharma Publications, 2017

The Rest And Repair Diet: Heal Your Gut, Improve Your Physical and Mental Health, and Lose Weight by Robert Keith Wallace, PhD, Samantha Wallace, Andrew Stenberg, MA, Jim Davis, DO, and Alexis Farley, Dharma Publications, 2019

Dharma Parenting: Understand Your Child's Brilliant Brain for Greater Happiness, Health, Success, and Fulfillment by Robert Keith Wallace, PhD, and Frederick Travis, PhD, Tarcher/Perigree, 2016

Transcendental Meditation and Maharishi AyurVeda

Science of Being and Art of Living: Transcendental Meditation by Maharishi Mahesh Yogi, MUM Press, Kindle edition, 2011

Maharishi Mahesh Yogi on the Bhagavad-Gita, A New Translation and Commentary, Chapters 1-6, MUM Press, 2016

One unbounded ocean of consciousness: Simple answers to the big questions in life by Dr Tony Nader, Aguilar, 2021

The Coherence Effect: Tapping into the Laws of Nature that Govern Health, Happiness, and Higher Brain Functioning by Robert Keith Wallace, PhD, Jay B. Marcus, and Chris S. Clark, MD, Armin Lear Press, 2020

Strength in Stillness: The Power of Transcendental Meditation by Bob Roth, Simon & Schuster, 2018

Catching the Big Fish: Meditation, Consciousness, and Creativity by David Lynch, Tarcher/Penguin 2007

An Introduction to Transcendental Meditation: Improve Your Brain Functioning, Create Ideal Health, and Gain Enlightenment Naturally, Easily, Effortlessly by Robert Keith Wallace, PhD, and Lincoln Akin Norton, Dharma Publications, 2016

Transcendental Meditation: A Scientist's Journey to Happiness, Health, and Peace, Adapted and Updated from The Physiology of Consciousness: Part 1 by Robert Keith Wallace, PhD, Dharma Publications, 2016

The Neurophysiology of Enlightenment: How the Transcendental Meditation and TM-Sidhi Program Transform the Functioning of the Human Body by Robert Keith Wallace, PhD, Dharma Publications, 2016

Maharishi Ayurveda and Vedic Technology: Creating Ideal Health for the Individual and World, Adapted and Updated from The Physiology of Consciousness: Part 2 by Robert Keith Wallace, PhD, Dharma Publications, 2016

In Balance leben: Wie wir trotz Stress mit unserer Energie richtig umgehen Broschiert (Translation: Living in Balance: How to deal with our energy properly despite stress) by Dr. med. Ulrich Bauhofer, Südwest Verlag, 2013

Business Performance

Success from Within: Discovering the Inner State that Creates Personal Fulfillment and Business Success by Jay B. Marcus, MIU Press, 1990

Enlightened Management: Building High-Performance People by Gerald Swanson and Bob Oates, MIU Press, 1987

Principles: Life and Work by Ray Dalio, Simon & Schuster, 2017

World-Class Brain by Harald Harung, PhD and Frederick Travis, PhD, Harvest, AS, 2019

Mindset: The New Psychology of Success by Carol S Dweck, Ballantine Books, 2007

Joy, Inc.: How We Built a Workplace People Love by Richard Sheridan,

Portfolio, 2013

Chief Joy Officer: How Great Leaders Elevate Human Energy and Eliminate Fear by Richard Sheridan, Portfolio, 2013

Recent Articles

Ma, X.; Yue, Z. Q.; Gong, Z. Q.; Zhang, H.; Duan, N. Y.; Shi, Y. T.; Wei, G. X.; & Li, Y. F. The Effect of Diaphragmatic Breathing on Attention, Negative Affect and Stress in Healthy Adults. Frontiers in psychology, 2017, 8, 874. https://doi.org/10.3389/fpsyg.2017.00874

Wallace, R.K. The Microbiome in Health and Disease from the Perspective of Modern Medicine and Ayurveda. Medicina 2020, 56, 462. doi: 10.3390/medicina56090462

Wallace, R.K. Ayurgenomics and Modern Medicine. Medicina 2020, 56, 661. doi: 10.3390/medicina56120661

Sharma, H.; Wallace, R.K. Ayurveda and Epigenetics. Medicina 2020, 56, 687. doi: 10.3390/medicina56120687

Wallace, R.K.; Wallace, T. Neuroadaptability and Habit: Modern Medicine and Ayurveda. Medicina 2021, 57, 90. doi: 10.3390/medicina57020090

Index

A

B

C

cortisol 46
creativity 15, 35, 58, 73, 96, 103, 156, 162

D

David Lynch Foundation viii, 187
DHARMIC 62, 63, 71, 101, 102, 103, 104, 105, 106, 108, 109
digestion 47, 84, 87, 121, 123, 124, 125, 126, 127, 128, 129, 150, 153, 167, 168,
        171, 176
dopamine 48

E

EEG 35, 51
Emotional Intelligence 25
emotional triggers 26
empathy 26, 35
endorphins 49
Energy State vii, 26, 27, 28, 59, 60, 61, 63, 64, 65, 66, 67, 68, 69, 73, 75, 76, 80,
        81, 83, 84, 85, 86, 87, 88, 89, 92, 101, 102, 103, 104, 105, 106, 108, 111,
        121, 122, 123, 124, 125, 126, 127, 129, 130, 131, 150, 153, 155, 156, 157,
        161, 162, 163, 164, 165, 168, 169, 171, 173, 175, 176, 183, 190
Energy State Quiz 26, 102, 105
Energy States 69, 129, 155, 163, 170, 175
enlightenment 52, 169
environment 151, 152
Environmental Coaching 84, 86
epigenetic 133
Essential Self vi, 6, 11, 29, 39, 43, 57
Evolve 39, 61
exercise 72, 80, 81, 86, 89, 102, 122, 123, 124, 127, 128, 130, 132, 134, 152,
        156, 157, 164, 165, 169, 171, 183
Experiment 39, 61, 81

F

fight or flight response 46

G

gene expression 47
Group Coaching 84, 86
Gut-Brain Axis viii, 71, 149

H

habit 28, 32, 35, 37, 48, 49, 57, 58, 59, 60, 61, 62, 63, 64, 71, 72, 73, 75, 76, 77, 79, 80, 81, 84, 85, 86, 91, 92, 93, 95, 102, 103, 104, 106, 108, 109, 111, 112, 151, 152, 153
Habit Map vii, 60, 71, 72, 73, 103, 105, 108, 152, 153
Habit Plan 72, 76, 81, 91, 103, 106, 152
habit stacking 77, 151
happiness 33, 34, 51, 130, 146, 147, 177, 187, 188
health ii, 26, 35, 43, 47, 51, 80, 83, 84, 108, 116, 126, 129, 139, 140, 141, 142, 145, 147, 149, 150, 153, 167, 168, 169, 183, 184, 185, 187
Health Coaching viii, 183
hippocampus 44, 45, 46, 47
hypothalamus 46

I

Improvement vii, 91
Integration vii, 91
intention 58, 72, 105, 152, 177, 185

J

James Clear 151, 190
journal 60, 85, 104

K

Kapha 27, 131, 132, 133, 170, 175, 176
Kathy 101, 107, 108, 109, 111, 112
keystone habits 33

L

Learn 31, 33, 59
Listen 31, 59

M

Maharishi AyurVeda 86, 184, 191
Maharishi International University 115, 116, 184
Maharishi Mahesh Yogi 52, 178, 191
Maharishi Mahesh Yogi, 52, 178, 191
Maintain Balance vii, 83, 104, 106, 109
Marshall Goldsmith 151

meditation 35, 51, 52, 137, 139, 140, 143, 145, 147, 156, 169
microbiome 43, 84, 132, 149, 150, 168
motivation 33, 34, 51, 130, 146, 147, 177, 187, 188
My Octopus Teacher 112

N

nervous system 5, 43, 44, 46, 138, 139, 149
neuroadaptability 5, 29, 35, 39, 48, 49, 51, 62, 86, 96, 113
Neuroplasticity 71
Neuroscience 40, 146
Neuro Self vi, 6, 29, 43, 57
noradrenalin 46

O

Outer Self vi, 6, 11, 12, 43, 57
oxytocin 49

P

parenting 76, 161, 162, 164
Paul 101, 104, 105, 106, 111, 112, 145, 188
P Energy State 27, 28, 59, 61, 63, 64, 67, 73, 75, 76, 80, 85, 88, 92, 104, 105,
    106, 122, 123, 125, 127, 131, 153, 156, 157, 163, 175, 176
performance 33, 34, 51, 130, 146, 147, 177, 187, 188
Personal Coaching 84
Pitta 27, 131, 132, 133, 170, 175, 176
PK Energy State 127
Prakriti 27, 130, 131, 133, 134
prefrontal cortex 45, 46, 47

Q

Quiet Indifference 73, 74, 93

R

recreation 14
relationships 5, 18, 23, 29, 37, 73, 76, 128
Rest and Repair Diet 33, 34, 51, 130, 146, 147, 177, 187, 188
rhythm vii, 79
Richard Sheridan 34

S

Y

yoga 33, 103, 108, 122, 169, 170

CPSIA information can be obtained
at www.ICGtesting.com
Printed in the USA
BVHW031523120521
607123BV00001B/30